LETTING GO OF OCD

LETTING GO

of OCD

OVERCOMING INTRUSIVE THOUGHTS,
REDUCING ANXIETY, AND
RECLAIMING YOUR LIFE

Zachary David Westerbeck

Published by OCD Space, Inc.

Paperback ISBN: 979-8-218-93912-0
Ebook ISBN: 979-8-218-93913-7

Cover and interior design by Liz Schreiter
Edited and produced by Reading List Editorial
ReadingListEditorial.com

Disclaimer

This book is not a substitute for medical advice, diagnosis, or treatment. It is intended for educational and informational purposes only.

Zach Westerbeck is not a licensed medical professional.

He is not trained in diagnosing psychological or medical conditions, and he is not a substitute for medical care or medical advice. If you require assistance with any mental health or medical issue, please contact your licensed health care provider. Only a qualified professional can provide an accurate diagnosis and determine the best course of treatment for your individual needs.

Zach Westerbeck makes no guarantees of any kind that the information or services provided will improve your situation.

While this book shares evidence-based strategies, tools, and personal experiences related to OCD recovery, every person's journey is unique. What works for one individual may not be appropriate for another.

If you are in crisis or need immediate support, contact your doctor, therapist, or a mental health crisis line in your area.

Your safety and well-being come first. Use the information in this book responsibly and always in partnership with professional care.

National Suicide Prevention Lifeline

If you or a loved one is experiencing thoughts of suicide or is in need of help, please call the 988 Lifeline.

CONTENTS

FOREWORD

I've been doing OCD work for more than a decade, and during that time I've treated many hundreds of people struggling with obsessive-compulsive disorder and clinical anxiety. I often tell patients, "No matter what's been happening for you, you're never going to tell me something I haven't heard before—probably many times." That's not because their experiences aren't painful or intense. It's because OCD is remarkably consistent in how it operates. After years in this field, there's very little about the disorder that surprises me anymore.

And after thousands of exposures, hundreds of cases, and years of treating OCD, here's what I'll tell you: Treating OCD is actually very simple.

Not easy. Simple.

By that, I don't mean there aren't important ideas to learn or skills that take time to practice. I mean that OCD is driven by a single, identifiable mechanism. Learning to interrupt that mechanism takes effort, repetition, and courage—but the underlying process itself is straightforward.

Over the years, I've developed little phrases and reminders to help patients keep their focus on what matters most. Things like, "If you pull the 'C' out of the OCD, your symptoms will unravel," or "Your OCD isn't happening to you—you're happening to your OCD." These aren't just catchy sayings. They're meant to anchor people when OCD tries to pull them back into familiar traps—reassurance-seeking, certainty-chasing, and compulsive problem-solving. OCD is very good at distracting you from the real work. Don't take the bait.

In 1966, Victor Meyer fundamentally changed our understanding of OCD when he demonstrated—empirically—that the disorder is maintained by compulsive behavior, not by the presence of intrusive thoughts themselves. OCD is a system, an engine, and compulsions are the fuel that keep it running. Trying to analyze, resolve, or neutralize intrusive thoughts only keeps that engine alive.

The analogy I often use is a mosquito bite. Scratching it may bring momentary relief, but it ultimately prolongs the itch. No amount of insight into why you want to scratch will make the itch stop. What changes the experience is resisting the urge to scratch—even while it's uncomfortable. Over time, the system settles. OCD works the same way.

This is why we say OCD is a behavioral problem. Compulsions are behaviors. Behaviors are choices. And choices, even difficult ones, can be changed. Getting better means learning to respond differently—again and again—until the system weakens. Simple. Not easy.

I myself live with OCD, which is where my belief that if you pull the "C" out of the OCD, the system begins to fall apart stems from. Zach Westerbeck knows that too. This book contains the strategies and tactics that will help pull away at that compulsive behavior so you can stop organizing your life around OCD and begin reclaiming it for yourself. *Letting Go of OCD* normalizes the full range of intrusive thoughts people are afraid to talk about, and it clearly explains what actually drives OCD and what doesn't. More importantly, it offers practical, step-by-step guidance rooted in evidence-based principles, without overcomplicating the process. Zach focuses on what matters most, drawing from both lived experience and clinical insight, and he does so with clarity, patience, and respect for the reader.

But there's another belief that Zach and I share: People don't necessarily need endless analysis or cathartic conversation to recover from OCD. What they need is a clear understanding of how the system works and consistent guidance in applying proven strategies in real time. That's why I've long believed that artificial intelligence—when grounded in evidence-based care—could play a meaningful role in helping people manage OCD more effectively. We already live much of our lives online—learning skills, managing our health, connecting with others, and solving problems in real time. Because OCD is a moment-to-moment behavioral disorder, AI-driven tools that can offer timely structure, reminders, and coaching when it matters most are particularly well-suited to support recovery.

That's why I'm so excited to see that Zach has gone beyond the excellent resources in this book to create OCD Space, and its AI OCD coach, Oscar. For those who want additional support applying these principles, Oscar exists as a practical extension— designed to help people practice skills, measure progress, and stay oriented toward recovery over time. Used well, it reinforces the same behavioral foundations that have guided effective OCD treatment for decades.

From where I stand, OCD Space and this book are part of an exciting moment—there are now more clinically reviewed, research-backed paths for recovering from OCD than ever. Whatever approach you're ready for, you can start treating your OCD now. It won't be easy, but—especially with the right tools— it can be simple.

—Chris J. K. Leins, MA, LPCC-S

PART 1

PREPARING FOR RECOVERY

INTRODUCTION

RECLAIMING YOUR LIFE FROM OCD

If you're reading this, there's a good chance you're tired—mentally, emotionally, maybe even physically. Tired of the thoughts that won't stop, the rituals that consume your time, and the fear that tells you that this might not ever get better.

I get it. I've been there too.

For years, OCD ruled my life. It convinced me I was broken, unsafe, and alone. It told me I was the only one having these disturbing thoughts, and that they must mean something about who I am. I lived in constant mental noise, shame, and fear. I want to tell you something I wish someone had told me earlier:

You are not alone. You are not your thoughts. And OCD recovery is 100 percent possible.

This book is not about achieving perfection or getting rid of every intrusive thought. It's about learning how to respond to OCD in a new way—one that gives you your life back. We'll talk about tools like the four core responses, exposure and response prevention (ERP), the letting go technique, and core mindset shifts that will help you build real momentum. We'll also explore how your lifestyle—your sleep, diet, exercise, meditation, and even how you use your phone—can support your healing.

My Story

My journey with OCD began in late 2015, when I was suddenly overwhelmed by intrusive thoughts that felt terrifying, real, and unfamiliar. I didn't know it was OCD; I just knew something felt deeply wrong. The fear, the rumination, and the shame consumed me. In 2016, I finally hit rock bottom and reached out for help. I was diagnosed with OCD and began formal therapy, including ERP, which is considered the gold standard for OCD treatment. ERP *did* help me start facing my fears and taking my life back.

But over time, I realized something important: ERP is essential, but it's not the whole picture. There were other pieces I had to figure out for myself, like how to manage my mindset, how to support my brain and body through lifestyle changes, and how to let go in real time when OCD came knocking. My hope with this book is to illuminate that larger picture. I want to give you all the tools I wish I'd had earlier so you can recover faster, feel more empowered, and start living the life you deserve.

You'll learn how to peel back the layers of OCD like an onion—gently, patiently, and with compassion. This process won't always be easy, but I promise you it will be worth it.

Everything I teach in this book, I live. These tools still support me every single day. OCD hasn't gone away completely, but it no longer runs my life. I want that same freedom for you.

You're not alone in this. I'll be here with you on every page.

1

WHAT TO EXPECT FROM THIS BOOK

When we're stuck in the OCD cycle, it can feel like we're trapped in our own mind with no map, no instructions, and no way out. We feel like prisoners. You might even be wondering right now if this book can really help you.

The answer is yes, and it's not just because it's full of proven tools and strategies. It's because this book is written by someone who's been in the trenches with you, who knows what it's like to live with OCD.

I'm not a psychologist. I'm not a researcher in a lab. I'm a real person who lives with OCD and who's spent years learning what actually works. I've done the formal therapy, I've studied the brain, I've worked with hundreds of clients, and I've lived through the darkest nights of fear, doubt, and hopelessness. What I'm sharing in this book is everything I wish I'd had when I was first diagnosed back in 2016.

If you've been searching for a step-by-step guide to help take your life back from OCD, this is it.

What This Book Will Help You Do

- Understand what OCD *really* is (not what pop culture or social media says it is)
- Learn the truth about intrusive thoughts and why they're junk content with no true meaning
- Break free from the compulsions that are secretly keeping you stuck
- Use tools like the four core responses, ERP, and the letting go technique to face fear and build emotional resilience
- Rewire your brain through helpful tools, mindset shifts, and daily lifestyle choices
- Build confidence, self-compassion, and momentum one small win at a time
- Create a sustainable, long-term recovery plan that actually works in the real world

How the Book Is Structured

I designed this book to follow the natural arc of the recovery journey. It's broken into seven parts:

1. **Preparing for Recovery:** We start by getting your mind in the right place. Think of this as putting on your mental armor and becoming an OCD warrior.
2. **Understanding OCD:** You'll learn how OCD works, why it sticks, and how it plays tricks on us.
3. **The Four Core Responses That Change Everything:** This tool is the foundation of OCD recovery. I'll teach you how to respond to OCD in ways that take its power away.
4. **Taking Action with ERP:** You'll learn exactly how to do exposure and response prevention, the gold standard treatment for OCD, and how to avoid the common pitfalls.

5. **Letting Go:** This powerful technique will teach you how to feel uncomfortable feelings and learn how to release them in a simple step-by-step process.

6. **Optimizing Your Brain and Body:** Your brain is an organ, and it needs support. Sleep, meditation, nutrition, exercise, supplements, nature, and even screen time all play a role in healing.

7. **Staying Free:** OCD recovery is possible, but it's also ongoing. I'll help you build a plan for staying free long after the book ends.

You don't need to read the whole book before getting started. In fact, I recommend that you take it chapter by chapter, apply what you're learning along the way, and come back to it often. Use it like a recovery playbook. Highlight it. Dog-ear the pages. Reread the sections that speak to you. This book is here to *work* for you.

A Few Promises Before We Begin

- I will be real with you. I'm not here to sugarcoat recovery, but I'll always leave you with hope.
- I will speak in plain, honest language—no confusing psych terms, no guilt, no judgment.
- I will remind you that you are not broken. Your brain is doing exactly what it was designed to do. It just needs a little rewiring.
- I will walk with you every step of the way. You are never alone on this journey.

This book is about reclaiming your life from OCD. It won't happen overnight. With the right tools, the right mindset, and a willingness to lean into discomfort, you can do this.

Let's get started.

A Quick Note on Getting Triggered

If you find yourself feeling triggered by something in this book—maybe even tempted to put it down and never return—I want you to know you're not alone. The same thing happened to me when I was starting my recovery journey.

I've written this book from the perspective of a fellow OCDer, and my intention is to be as gentle and supportive as possible. Sometimes just reading about OCD can stir things up. If that happens, I encourage you to stick with it. Take a breath, take a break if you need to, and come back when you're ready.

The information in these pages has the power to set you free. You're stronger than you think, and you're never alone on this path.

Take the Next Step with OCD Space

This book is your road map to OCD recovery. Read it, use it, live it. You don't have to do this perfectly, just consistently. Progress over perfection. Always.

OCD doesn't wait for you to flip to the right chapter. It can hit when it's two in the morning and you're alone with your thoughts. Back in 2016, I learned firsthand how terrifying and isolating those moments can feel. I know that's when support matters most.

That's why I built OCD Space and Oscar—our clinically trained AI OCD coach—to be the tool I wish I had. Oscar can help you apply recovery skills in real time, when OCD feels loud and overwhelming.

Start your free trial at OCDspace.com

Membership is HSA/FSA eligible

2

THE MINDSETS THAT WILL SET YOU FREE

Before we dive into tools like the four core responses, ERP, or the letting go technique, we need to talk about something even more important: your mindset.

When I started recovery, I wanted someone to give me a script and just tell me what to do to feel better. What I didn't realize was that how I *thought* about OCD, discomfort, and healing was the real starting point.

OCD recovery isn't about doing things perfectly. It's about how we show up when things feel messy, hard, or uncertain.

These are the ten mental shifts I had to make, and I still use them to this day. If you can start practicing these, even just a little bit, I promise your recovery will feel more doable.

1. Nothing Else Matters More Right Now

When we're deep in the OCD cycle, it's easy to focus on everything *except* what we actually need: healing. You might be trying to keep up with work, school, relationships, fitness, or some version of your "old self."

Here's the tough truth: You can't fully enjoy any of those things until you take care of your brain.

Back in 2016, I kept telling myself I could push through. That if I just got promoted, worked out more, or fixed my sleep, the OCD would go away. It didn't. My brain was begging for help, and I was ignoring it.

Your number one priority right now is reclaiming your life from OCD. Everything else can wait. This is your foundation.

2. Stop Hoping OCD Will Just Go Away

This one hit me hard in the early days. I thought I could just ignore OCD and tuck it into a corner of my life. I tried to pretend it wasn't there and hoped it would eventually disappear.

But OCD doesn't work like that.

The more I avoided it, the stronger it got. The more I tried to live my life *around* OCD, the more it boxed me in. It wasn't until I stopped running, embraced my reality, and finally said, "Okay, this is what I'm dealing with, now what can I do about it?" that things actually started to change.

You don't have to love OCD. You just have to stop pretending it's not there. That's when real recovery begins.

3. Buy In—Even If You're Skeptical

You might be thinking, "Sure, this worked for Zach and other people, but what if it doesn't work for me?"

I get that. I was skeptical too. Being skeptical or doubtful is actually a part of living with OCD. You don't need to deny the doubt; embrace it. But also recognize that OCD wants you to be doubtful so that you don't use the tools I'm going to teach you in this book.

Truthfully, it wasn't until I committed—*really* committed—to the process that things started to change. I had to go all-in before I saw any results.

So if you're here, reading this, I want to challenge you to do the same. Don't just skim the pages. Show up and use the tools.

The more you invest in this process, the more it will give back to you.

4. Embrace Uncertainty

OCD wants you to believe that the *only* way to feel safe is to be 100 percent certain.

- What if I'm a bad person?
- What if I'm just in denial about who I truly am?
- What if this thought means something about me?

These questions feel like emergencies, but they're actually false alarms. Recovery means learning to sit with these questions *without needing answers*.

The more you practice saying, "Maybe, maybe not," the more your brain learns that uncertainty is safe. More on this later.

5. Tolerate Discomfort

There's no way around this: OCD recovery will be uncomfortable at times. But discomfort is not danger.

When I finally accepted that feeling anxious didn't mean I was unsafe—that it was just a sensation—I was able to stop running from it. Over time, anxiety lost its power over me.

Healing happens when we stop trying to *get rid of* the feelings and start learning to *ride them out*.

6. Trust the Process

Recovery isn't linear. Some days you'll feel unstoppable. Others, it'll feel like you're back at square one. That's normal.

OCD will try to convince you it's not working. It'll say, "This time is different." That's just another trick.

Stick with it. Use the tools. Keep showing up. It's working, even when it doesn't feel like it.

7. Just Do Today

OCD recovery can feel overwhelming if you try to figure it all out at once.

You might think, "What if I can't do this forever? How will I keep this up for years? What if this stops working?"

It's not your job to solve those questions.

Your job is to just do today. To just read one page of this book. To show up for the next exposure. To make one accepting response. To resist one compulsion.

If you focus on doing recovery well for just today, the future takes care of itself.

"Win the day. Stack enough of those, and you win your life."

8. Be Willing to Do the Work

OCD recovery isn't something that just magically happens. It's something you actively participate in. That means you have to be willing to face fear, lean into discomfort, and show up for yourself even when every part of you wants to avoid it.

Willingness is the difference maker. Over the years, I've coached so many people through this process, and one of the biggest indicators of whether someone is ready to reclaim their life is this: They're *willing*. Willing to feel anxiety. Willing to stop compulsions. Willing to let go of needing certainty and start living anyway.

You don't have to feel brave. You don't have to feel confident. You just have to be *willing* to take one small step, even if your voice shakes and your hands are sweaty.

9. You Don't Have to Do This Perfectly

OCD will even try to turn recovery into an obsession, telling you that you need to do ERP *just right*, say the accepting statement *exactly right*, or feel *perfectly okay* after doing an exposure.

That's not the goal.

The goal is to show up as best you can with the tools and energy you have in the moment.

You're allowed to be human. You're allowed to feel messy. You're allowed to get it "wrong" sometimes.

If you're doing recovery, 85 percent to 90 percent of the time, you're doing amazing.

Perfectionism feeds OCD. Acceptance of imperfection sets us free.

10. Know Your "Why"

When things get hard—and they will—you need something to hold on to.

- Who are you doing this for?
- What has OCD taken from you?
- What do you want to get back?

For me, it was my peace of mind. My relationships with my wife, family, friends, and future children. My ability to be present. Your "why" will anchor you when everything else feels shaky.

We'll talk more about this in the next chapter, but start thinking about it now. Write it down. Keep it close.

It's Your Turn

Take a few minutes to write these mindsets down in your OCD journal. Keep them somewhere you'll see them often. When things feel hard, come back to them.

Key Takeaway

Mindset is the foundation of recovery. You don't need to feel ready; you just need to be willing. Lean into uncertainty. Welcome discomfort. Trust the process. Remember why you're doing this.

3

WHAT IS YOUR WHY?

There's a reason you're reading this book.

Maybe OCD has taken away your peace of mind. Maybe it's stolen your ability to be present with your partner, your kids, your friends. Maybe it's held you back from showing up at work, or saying yes to travel, or enjoying the simple things in life without being dragged into mental chaos.

Whatever it is—you want your life back.

That's your *why*.

In recovery, our why becomes our anchor. It's what we come back to on the hard days when we're doing ERP, our anxiety is screaming, and OCD is throwing every "what-if" in the book at us. When it would be easier to avoid the fear and fall back into old habits, we remember our *why* to keep pushing forward.

Why This Matters

Recovery isn't about chasing perfection. It's about choosing meaning over comfort. Choosing action over avoidance. Choosing the life we want while feeling uncomfortable emotions.

To keep choosing that—especially when things get uncomfortable—we have to remember what's at stake.

Values-Based Living: The Deeper Why

OCD recovery isn't just about getting rid of anxiety; it's about reclaiming the life we want to live. That's where values-based living comes in.

Our values are the things that matter to us the most: spending quality time with our partner, friends, or parents; growing in our career or studies; being creative, adventurous, kind, inquisitive, connected—whatever lights us up.

Values-based living invites us to take actions that align with the people, places, and things that matter to us most, even when it's uncomfortable or scary.

When we root our recovery in our values, ERP and the other tools in this book become more than just techniques. They become choices to show up for ourselves, our dreams, and our people regardless of what OCD throws our way.

For example, I value deep connection with my wife, children, family, and friends. It became much easier to do OCD recovery when I realized OCD was trying to take something away from me that I valued deeply and wanted back.

Anchoring yourself in your values as you go on this journey is one of the most important things you can do. Please keep this in mind as you work your way through the rest of this book, and remind yourself of your values.

Take a moment and ask yourself these questions:

- What are my values?
- What do I care about more than certainty?
- What has OCD taken from me?
- What do I want to reclaim in my life?

- Who am I doing this for?
- What does my ideal life look like even with OCD still in the background?

Be honest with yourself. If the answers feel blurry right now, that's okay. Just take your best guess. Put pen to paper and see what comes out. It's okay if your brain tries to overanalyze it.

For me, my why was simple: I wanted peace. I wanted to be present with the people I loved, including my wife, children, parents, sister, and friends because connection with others is what I value. That vision pulled me forward when nothing else could.

And now? My life isn't perfect, but it's mine, and I'm proud of it. That's what I want for you too.

It's Your Turn

Take five minutes right now and write about your *why* in your OCD journal. Why do you want recovery? What kind of life are you fighting for?

Keep it simple. Put pen to paper and see what comes out. Let this be your compass when the path feels hard.

Key Takeaway

Recovery can feel challenging, but it's worth it because of your *why*. Take time to name it. Write it down. Speak it out loud. Keep it close. It will carry you further than willpower ever could.

PART 2

UNDERSTANDING OCD

4

WHAT OCD REALLY IS

Let's clear something up right now: OCD isn't about being neat or organized.

It's not about color-coded planners or washing our hands a few extra times. It's not a personality quirk. It's not something cute to say when you like your pantry a certain way.

OCD is a real, misunderstood brain health challenge that impacts our thoughts, emotions, and behavior, and it can be very disruptive when left untreated.

When you live with OCD, you're not just dealing with "worry." You're stuck in a cycle of terrifying, intrusive thoughts paired with compulsive behaviors that feel *necessary* to keep something bad from happening or to feel like a good person. These behaviors don't feel optional. They feel urgent, all-consuming, and high-stakes.

The truth is that OCD is a disorder of doubt and fear, and it attacks what matters most to us.

You're Not Alone

According to the World Health Organization, it's estimated that anywhere from 80 to 320 million people worldwide live with OCD. That's up to one adult in forty. And those are just the reported numbers.[1]

Let that sink in. If you feel isolated or ashamed, I want you to know this: You're not alone—not even close. I know this is true because I speak to people around the world when they DM me on social media from different countries and cultures struggling with the same thoughts and emotions.

Millions of us are living through the same cycle of fear, doubt, and compulsions. The difference is that you're here, learning how to break it.

What Does OCD Actually Look Like?

Here's what typically happens when we're stuck in the OCD loop:

1. An intrusive thought shows up (usually unwanted, uncomfortable, or disturbing).
2. We attach a negative meaning. ("This thought is bad.")
3. We feel a rush of anxiety, shame, or guilt.
4. Our brain screams, "Fix this. Figure it out. Make it go away. Do something!"
5. We perform a compulsion (mental or physical) to get relief.
6. We feel temporary relief—until the next thought hits.

Around and around we go.

I'll break this down more in the next few chapters, but for now, just know this: OCD feeds on our desire to feel certain, safe, and morally good.

It's not about the content of our thoughts. It's about our reaction to them.

"But My Thoughts Feel So Real"

I used to think I was the only person in the world having the thoughts I was having.

Back in 2015, when my OCD first showed up, it wasn't about handwashing or checking locks. It was about my sexual orientation. Thoughts flooded my brain out of nowhere: "What if you're actually gay and just in denial?" My heart would pound, my stomach would drop, and I'd spiral into hours of compulsions—Googling, mentally reviewing past experiences, analyzing how I felt around certain people.

I wasn't homophobic—I deeply respect all orientations. But I had always identified as straight, and suddenly I was experiencing thoughts that felt disconnected from who I truly believed I was. It wasn't about judgment; it was about my identity. I was desperate for certainty.

That's what OCD does. It latches on to what matters most to us and says, "What if?"

- What if I snap and hurt someone?
- What if I did something awful and forgot?
- What if this thought means I'm a bad person?
- What if I've been in denial my whole life?

OCD doesn't care what the theme is. It cares about our reaction. The harder I tried to make the thoughts go away, the louder they got.

Why OCD Is Called "the Doubting Disorder"

People often call OCD "the doubting disorder" because it can create chronic, painful uncertainty. You might feel like you can't trust your thoughts, your memories, your feelings, or even your identity.

OCD will always ask for more:

- More certainty
- More reassurance
- One last check
- One more Google search
- One final confession

Here's the kicker: We will never actually get the certainty we're looking for. OCD is a trap that promises relief and delivers more anxiety.

What's Going On in Our Brain?

I'm not going to overload you with neuroscience, but here's a simplified version of what's happening behind the scenes:

1. Our brain perceives a threat (even if it's not real).
2. It sends out a fear signal: "This is dangerous—fix it!"
3. We do something (a mental or physical compulsion) to reduce the fear.
4. That compulsion reinforces the fear, teaching our brain: "Good job! You survived because you did that thing."
5. Now our brain thinks it needs to do that thing every time the fear shows up.

It's like a fire alarm going off every time we make toast. There's no real fire, but our brain reacts like the house is burning down.

This cycle keeps repeating until we change our response.

You Are Not Your Thoughts

If you remember one thing from this chapter, let it be this:

*You are not your thoughts. But how
you respond to them matters.*

Everyone has weird, random, even disturbing thoughts sometimes. People without OCD can shrug them off. But if you have OCD, those thoughts feel sticky. Meaningful. Dangerous. They feel like emergencies.

Here's the wild part: Science backs this up.

In a study led by Dr. Adam Radomsky at Concordia University,[2] researchers asked both people with and without OCD to report on the kinds of thoughts they experienced. Nearly all participants, regardless of diagnosis, reported having intrusive thoughts—including ones about harming loved ones, acting out sexually, or questioning their identity.

The only difference? People with OCD felt immense guilt, anxiety, and urgency around those thoughts, and they responded to them with compulsions. The non-OCD group didn't give the thoughts meaning. They just moved on.

That's the key. It's not the presence of the thought—it's the reaction to it. OCD trains your brain to *overreact* to junk thoughts like they're life-and-death situations.

So let me say it again: We are not our thoughts. We are how we respond to them.

The best part is that our response is something we can learn to change. More on this in upcoming chapters.

Labeling Thoughts Negatively

One last thing before we move on: In the beginning, you might hear me describe intrusive thoughts as *weird*, *disturbing*, or *horrible*, and I do that because that's how they feel at first. That's how I described them when I was in it. But as we go deeper into recovery, I want to invite you to start changing that language.

Here's why: When we label thoughts as "bad" or "wrong," we reinforce the fear around them. The brain learns to think, "This is dangerous. Pay attention!" OCD feeds off that.

Over time, the goal is to see these thoughts as what they really are: neutral noise. Mental junk. Just thoughts. They don't need a label. They just need to be allowed to come and go on their own time like passing clouds in the sky.

We'll get more into this mindset shift soon. But for now, just know this: It's not about what the thought says; it's about how we show up in response. That's where our power is.

Understanding the Power of Externalization

OCD can feel deeply personal.

The thoughts it sends often sound like our own voice. They show up in our tone, using our fears and targeting the things that matter most to us.

But here's the truth: You are not your thoughts. And you are not your OCD.

To help make that distinction clearer, we use a technique called externalization.

It comes from narrative therapy, and it's been shown to help people with OCD. Here's what it does:

- Reduces shame
- Creates distance from intrusive thoughts

- Helps people take more effective, values-aligned action

Externalization means giving your OCD a separate identity from yourself. Your OCD is not you. It is the overactive, fear-driven part of your brain trying to keep you safe but doing it in unnecessary ways.

So, try giving it a name.

Why a Neutral Name Matters

When choosing a name like, we should be intentionally picking something neutral or even playful.

Why?

Because if we name the OCD something like Idiot, Monster, or Demon, we unintentionally teach our brain that our thoughts are dangerous, horrible, or something to fear.

That just keeps the OCD cycle alive.

By giving it a name that's a little lighter—something like Irving, Stanley, or even Doris—we remind ourselves this is just the fear voice. It's not evil. It's just confused.

That shift helps our brain soften its response and stop reinforcing that thoughts are threats.

A Neuroscience Perspective

Externalization isn't just a mindset trick. It's rooted in how the brain actually works.

Intrusive thoughts come from deeper brain regions tied to emotion, threat detection, and habit loops, not from the prefrontal cortex, which is responsible for logic, reasoning, and decision-making.

In other words, you didn't *choose* the thought. You didn't *create* it. It bubbled up automatically from regions you're not responsible for.

So when we say, "That's just Arnold, my OCD," we're honoring a very real neurological distinction in the brain.

Language That Shifts Everything

Instead of saying, "I'm having a horrible thought," say, "Peter is being loud right now" or "That's just Susan doing what Susan does," or "Fritz is playing the 'what if' game again."

It's a small shift, but it's a powerful one.

Recovery doesn't require controlling your OCD. It requires learning how to respond to it differently. More on this later.

Backed by Research

Research supports this approach.[3] Externalizing OCD thoughts has been shown to help reduce fusion (overidentifying with thoughts), increase treatment engagement, and empower individuals to act more compassionately toward themselves.

This is especially important because so many of us with OCD carry shame. We think, "What does it mean that I'm thinking this?" or "Does this say something about who I am?"

When we say, "That's just my OCD doing what my OCD does," we're reminding ourselves this is a disorder, not a reflection of our character.

The Trap to Avoid: "Is This OCD or Is This Me?"

One of the sneakiest tricks OCD plays is making us question our own mind. You might find yourself wondering, "Is this an OCD thought or a me thought?"

It's a totally understandable question, but it's also a trap.

The more we try to figure that out, the more we're stuck in analysis. That question becomes a compulsion—an attempt to feel certain, safe, and morally clean.

So here's your new mindset: "If I'm asking whether it's OCD—it probably is. And I don't need to solve it."

We respond the same way to all sticky thoughts. With acceptance. With indifference. With a shoulder shrug. We'll be talking more about these helpful responses in the coming chapters.

Key Takeaway

We're stuck in OCD's game the moment we ask, "Is this OCD or is this me?"

We don't need to figure it out. We just need to learn to respond differently.

Take the Next Step with OCD Space

OCD recovery doesn't just happen while you're reading a book; it happens in the moments OCD shows up in real life.

OCD Space is a digital recovery platform where you can work with Oscar, our clinically trained AI OCD coach, 24/7. Oscar will help guide you through OCD recovery so you can keep making progress anytime, anywhere.

Join OCDspace.com and start working with Oscar today

5

WHY DO I HAVE OCD?

This is one of the first questions people ask when they're diagnosed with OCD: Why me?

It's a fair question. While there's no single answer, there is a helpful way to understand what's going on—one that moves you out of guilt and into action.

The truth is that OCD isn't our fault. We didn't choose this. We didn't manifest it by having "bad" thoughts or being a certain kind of person. OCD is the result of a few key factors coming together, and once we understand those, we can start working with our brain instead of against it.

1. Brain Wiring and Genetics

Let's start with the basics: OCD is a brain-based disorder.

Research shows that OCDers have differences in how our brains process fear, uncertainty, and emotional regulation. Specifically, our brain's "threat detection system" tends to be overactive, including in areas like the almond-shaped amygdala and the anterior cingulate cortex. That means our brain might send out danger signals even when there's no real danger.

Think of it like this: Our brain's fire alarm is going off because we burned toast, but it's reacting like the whole house is on fire.

Beyond that, neuroscience has identified a specific brain circuit that plays a major role in OCD symptoms: the cortico-striato-thalamo-cortical (CSTC) loop.

This loop is responsible for regulating thoughts and movement as well as filtering information. In people with OCD, this circuit becomes overactive and "sticky," which makes it harder for the brain to let go of unwanted thoughts or disengage from compulsions.

One study published in *Neuropsychopharmacology*[4] showed that hyperconnectivity in the CSTC loop—especially between the orbitofrontal cortex and the striatum—was strongly associated with compulsive behaviors in OCD.

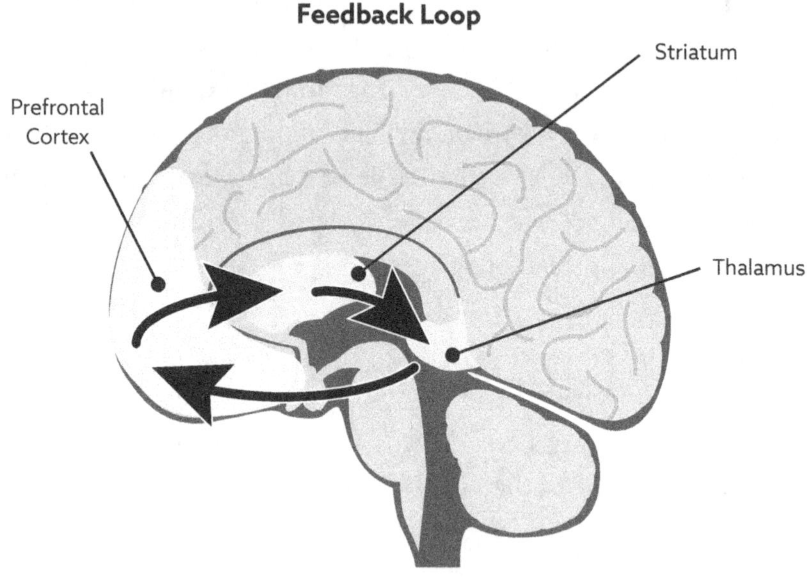

On top of that, there's often a genetic component. If someone in your family struggles with anxiety, OCD, or related conditions, it increases the likelihood that you might too. It's not guaranteed—but it can be part of the picture, as supported by an article in the *Indian Journal of Psychiatry*.[5]

OCD isn't a moral failing—it's a neurological and psychological condition. And like any condition, it can be treated.

2. Early Life Experiences

Many people with OCD grew up in environments that emphasized the following:

- High expectations
- Control or perfectionism
- Moral or religious rigidity
- Shame around certain thoughts or behaviors

Sometimes trauma is involved, and sometimes it's more subtle, like growing up in a home where mistakes weren't tolerated or emotions weren't safe to express.

None of this means your parents or caregivers intentionally caused your OCD. But it *can* help explain why your brain may have learned to associate certain thoughts with danger, shame, or urgency.

OCD loves to latch on to fear, especially fears that were modeled or reinforced early in life.

3. Stress and Life Transitions

In many people (myself included), OCD shows up or ramps up during times of major stress or life transitions, like starting college, moving, becoming a parent, dealing with illness, transitioning in your career, or going through a breakup.

In late 2015, I was navigating a high-stress period of my life, and, out of nowhere, I started having intrusive thoughts that completely wrecked me. It felt like my brain broke overnight.

In hindsight, I can see that the stress had been building. My nervous system was already overwhelmed. When OCD showed up, my brain latched on to the content of the thoughts as if they were emergencies.

Stress doesn't cause OCD on its own, but it often is the trigger if you're already predisposed.

4. It's Not Our Fault, but It Is Our Responsibility

I know this can feel heavy. I want you to hear me clearly: You didn't choose OCD. You're not weak. You're not broken.

But now that you know what it is—and how it works—you do have a choice: Keep reacting to OCD the way you always have or learn a new response that sets you free.

That's what this book is about.

When "Why Do I Have OCD?" Becomes a Trap

For many people with OCD, *"Why do I have OCD?"* becomes one of the most obsessive questions of all. And it makes sense—when we're suffering, our brain wants an explanation.

But here's the problem: This question often turns into a **mental compulsion.**

Some OCDers get stuck analyzing their past, trying to connect dots, and searching for the "root cause," hoping that if they can just figure it out, they'll finally feel relief. But OCD doesn't get solved by understanding *why* it exists—it gets weakened by changing how we respond to it.

Even if we found the perfect answer, it wouldn't stop intrusive thoughts or break the cycle. The only way to do that is with new behaviors: learning to recognize compulsions, resisting reassurance, and using the other tools you'll learn in this book.

So if you catch yourself spiraling with the "why" question, remind yourself: **"Maybe I'll never know exactly why I have OCD. And that's okay. My job is to recover anyway."**

Key Takeaway

We have OCD because of how our brains are wired, how we've learned to respond to fear, and how stress shaped our system. It's not our fault. Recovery becomes possible the moment we take ownership of what happens next.

Are you willing and ready to take ownership of your recovery?

6

OBSESSIONS

THE PAIN OF UNCERTAINTY

Since you live with OCD, you know this already: Intrusive thoughts can feel terrifying.

They show up out of nowhere, often relating to the things we care most deeply about. They bring a heavy emotional punch filled with anxiety, fear, guilt, shame, and disgust. Even though they're just thoughts, they don't *feel* like "just thoughts."

That's because OCD starts thoughts with "What if . . .?"

What Are Obsessions?

Obsessions are unwanted, intrusive thoughts, images, impulses, or sensations that create a feeling of fear or distress. They feel important, urgent, and high-stakes. They're almost always centered around uncertainty.

The thoughts themselves aren't dangerous, but our reactions to them (trying to get certainty, trying to "figure them out," trying to avoid feeling bad) are what fuel the OCD cycle. Obsessions are

OCD's way of saying, "Hey . . . are you *sure* you're safe? Are you *sure* you're a good person? Better double-check."

Just to be clear—*everyone* has unusual thoughts sometimes. The difference with OCD is that the thoughts feel *sticky*. We don't just shrug them off. We analyze them, ruminate on them, try to solve them, and that's what pulls us deeper into the loop.

Common OCD Subtypes (with Examples)

This list below is not exhaustive, but these are some of the most common OCD subtypes I've seen among hundreds of clients. You might resonate with one—or several. That's normal. OCD loves to change things up and see what else he can bother us with. When OCD switches it up, we call it the OCD Ninja.

This is important: Just because a thought feels disturbing doesn't mean it's true. The themes OCD chooses usually go after the things we care about most, like our identity, our safety, our values, and our loved ones.

Here are some common OCD subtypes, along with examples of intrusive thoughts that may show up in each.

Contamination OCD

- "What if I touched something dangerous and now I'll get sick—or make someone else sick?"
- "What if I didn't wash my hands well enough and I spread germs?"

This subtype is often focused on dirt, illness, chemicals, or other perceived contaminants.

Just Right/Perfectionism OCD

- "What if I didn't say that sentence exactly right and something bad happens?"
- "If I don't do this ritual the 'right' number of times, I'll feel off or incomplete."

The goal here isn't always safety—it's about getting rid of the feeling that something is "off" or that something bad will happen.

Relationship OCD (ROCD)

- "What if I don't actually love my partner?"
- "What if I'm secretly not attracted to them and I'm leading them on?"

This subtype targets our connection with loved ones—especially romantic partners—and causes doubt.

Sexual Orientation OCD (SO-OCD)

- "What if I'm actually gay and don't know it?"
- "What if I'm actually straight but secretly hiding it from myself?"

This isn't about homophobia—it's about intense fear of not knowing who we truly are.

Pedophilia OCD (POCD)

- "What if I'm attracted to children?"
- "Why did I notice that kid's body? Does that mean something?"

These thoughts can feel horrifying for the person experiencing them. They don't reflect real intent—they reflect fear.

Harm OCD

- "What if I suddenly lose control and stab someone?"
- "What if I ran someone over and didn't realize it?"

This subtype creates intense fear of hurting others even when we would never want to.

Scrupulosity OCD

- "What if I offended God without realizing it?"
- "What if I committed an unforgivable sin and I'm going to hell?"

This theme attacks religious or moral beliefs, often rooted in fear of being immoral or impure.

Existential OCD

- "What if none of this is real?"
- "What if I'm living in a simulation and nothing matters?"

This one spirals into deep philosophical questions and a desperate need for an answer.

Health OCD

- "What if this headache is actually a brain tumor?"
- "What if the doctor missed something serious?"

Those of us with health OCD often compulsively check symptoms, seek reassurance, or overly research medical information.

Real Event OCD

- "What if that mistake I made years ago means I'm a horrible person?"
- "What if I actually hurt someone and forgot about it?"

This subtype fixates on past events—often real but minor mistakes—and spins them into moral crises.

False Memory OCD

- "What if I did something terrible and I just don't remember?"
- "What if I cheated and my brain is hiding it from me?"

This subtype centers around the fear that we did something wrong in the past and our brain is hiding or misremembering it.

What All Obsessions Have in Common

No matter the subtype, obsessions tend to do the following:

- Feel intrusive and unwanted
- Cause anxiety, doubt, or guilt
- Create a sense of urgency ("I have to figure this out!")
- Feel "sticky"—you can't stop thinking about them
- Attack what you care about most

Here's something important you need to hear: Just because you're not having an intense emotional reaction every time—or even if you've done something in the past that feels similar to your feared thought—that does not mean you don't have OCD.

It doesn't make you a terrible person. We are human and imperfect. We all make mistakes we sometimes wish we could change. OCD will find anything that feels close enough to hook us in. OCD loves to distort the past and twist facts into fear.

In reality, OCD latches on to whatever we care about and whatever we give meaning to. While we just covered many common subtypes, this list is by no means exhaustive. OCD can attach itself to *anything* that triggers fear, doubt, or uncertainty.

That might sound intimidating at first, but here's an empowering fact: No matter what the thought is, the way we respond to OCD is always the same. That's exactly what we're going to unpack in the rest of this book.

Key Takeaway

Obsessions are intrusive thoughts that trigger fear, shame, sadness, or guilt. They're not dangerous—but they feel that way. OCD will use whatever topic gets our attention, but the solution is always the same: how we respond.

7

COMPULSIONS

THE SNEAKY WAYS WE STAY STUCK

Now you know what obsessions are—those sticky, fear-filled thoughts that trigger anxiety, shame, sadness, or dread. If obsessions are the spark, compulsions are the fuel.

Compulsions are the things we do—mentally or physically—to try to feel better, get certainty, or make the discomfort go away. While they might give us relief in the moment, they're the exact thing keeping us stuck in the OCD cycle.

Let me say that again, because it's huge: Compulsions are the oxygen keeping OCD alive.

The only reason OCD keeps showing up with the same junk thoughts is because somewhere along the way, your brain learned that reacting to them gave you relief. That relief is temporary, and it trains your brain to keep seeing the thought as a threat.

Common Types of Compulsions

Compulsions come in many forms. Some are super obvious. Others are so sneaky we don't even realize we're doing them. Here are the most common categories.

Avoidance

We may avoid people, places, objects, or situations that might trigger a scary thought or uncomfortable feeling. Here's what this can look like:

- Not watching certain shows for fear they'll trigger harm or sexual thoughts
- Avoiding knives or sharp objects
- Refusing to drive past certain areas
- Skipping social events because of OCD "what-ifs"

Avoidance is a compulsion. You're still responding to the fear and giving it meaning.

Checking

We may engage in physical or mental checking to make sure something bad didn't happen (or won't happen). Here's what this can look like:

- Checking locks or appliances repeatedly
- Mentally reviewing past actions: "Did I touch that person inappropriately?"
- Scanning your body for groinal responses or anxiety levels
- Rereading texts to make sure you didn't offend someone

Mental Review

We might go back over memories, feelings, or imagined scenarios to "figure it out." Here's what this can look like:

- Asking "What did I feel in that moment?"
- Wondering "Did I like the thought?"
- Thinking "How did I react to that person?"
- Questioning "Was my attraction real or fake?"

This one is super common in relationship OCD, SO-OCD, harm OCD, POCD, and real event OCD.

Reassurance-Seeking

We might ask others or ourselves for confirmation that everything is "okay." Here's what this can look like:

- Asking "Do you think I would actually do that?"
- Googling symptoms, conditions, or experiences
- Asking your partner "Are you sure you love me?"
- Reading Reddit threads or forums to see if someone else had the same thought

Mental or Physical Rituals

We might do or say things to "cancel out" a thought or prevent something bad from happening. Here's what this can look like:

- Praying repeatedly to neutralize a fear
- Repeating phrases or numbers
- Touching items in a certain way or order
- Counting, tapping, or mentally "erasing" bad images

Confessing

We might confess something over and over to get relief or avoid guilt. Here's what this can look like:

- Feeling compelled to tell someone about a thought you had
- Repeating events to a partner or friend to see how they react
- Bringing up past behavior to get reassurance that you're still a good person

Emotional Checking

We might check how we feel to "prove" or "disprove" something OCD is saying. Here's what this can look like:

- Thinking "If I feel anxious, it must mean the thought is real."
- Deciding "If I don't feel guilty, maybe I liked it."
- Thinking "If I don't feel love right now, maybe I'm with the wrong person."
- Concluding "If I don't feel anxious, it means I liked the thought all along."

Emotional checking is a sneaky compulsion. OCD turns our feelings into "evidence." Sometimes anxiety doesn't come after a thought—it shows up first. And then OCD jumps in and tells us, "The fact that you feel anxious must mean something," or "If you don't feel guilty, that must mean you liked it." In these moments, the emotion becomes the trigger, and checking how we feel becomes the compulsion. Either way, the cycle is the same: Discomfort shows up, and OCD pushes us to check for certainty.

Thought Blocking

This is one of the more subtle mental compulsions, and it can feel helpful in the moment. Thought blocking happens when we try to force a thought out of our mind as soon as it appears. Here's what this can look like:

- Commanding ourselves to "Stop thinking about that."
- Thinking "Go away, thought."
- Deciding "I'm not allowed to think that."
- Distracting ourselves with "I need to think really hard about something else."

It can also show up as physically tensing, distracting ourselves, or mentally yelling "no" to try to stop the thought from continuing.

Here's the problem: The more we resist a thought, the more it sticks. When we try to block a thought, we're telling our brain, "This is dangerous. This isn't allowed." That only reinforces the fear and keeps OCD loud.

Rumination: The Compulsion You Can't See

Rumination is one of the most common compulsions in OCD—and one of the more challenging to stop because it feels like we're doing something productive. It's not like checking a stove or washing hands. It happens quietly in our mind.

Rumination is when we repeatedly think about a thought, feeling, memory, or hypothetical scenario, trying to get certainty, relief, or an answer. It's the mental version of checking. We replay things. We analyze. We debate. We try to "figure it out." We search for the perfect conclusion that finally makes us feel calm.

The reality is that **rumination is not problem solving. Rumination is a ritual.**

And every time we ruminate, we teach the brain, *"This thought matters. This thought is dangerous. Keep analyzing it."* That's how OCD stays alive.

How to Know You're Ruminating

A simple way to know you're ruminating is to ask yourself:

- Am I trying to get certainty?
- Am I trying to feel relief?
- Am I trying to prove or disprove something?
- Am I trying to "solve" the thought so I can finally move on?

If the answer is yes, it's probably rumination.

Why Rumination Feels So Urgent

OCD makes rumination feel necessary. It tells us:

- "You need to figure this out right now."
- "This thought means something."
- "If you don't solve it, you're irresponsible."
- "You won't be able to relax until you get clarity."

But clarity is the trap. OCD doesn't want the answer—it wants the ritual.

How to Stop Ruminating (The Simple Method)

Stopping rumination isn't about forcing the thought away. It's about refusing to engage with it.

Here's what to do:

1. **Label it immediately:** "This is rumination."
2. **Allow discomfort:** "This feeling is uncomfortable, but I can handle it."

3. **Refuse the debate:** No analyzing, no reviewing, no mental checking.
4. **Return to your life:** Shift your attention to what you were doing before OCD pulled you in.

At first, it will feel like you're ignoring something important. That's normal. That's the withdrawal. That's your brain learning that it doesn't need to solve every thought.

The Most Important Reminder

If you stop ruminating and anxiety spikes, it doesn't mean you did the wrong thing. It means you stopped the ritual.

That discomfort is a sign you're doing recovery correctly.

Compulsions Feel Like Safety, but They're a Trap

Compulsions give us that hit of relief in the moment—like an exhale after a panic attack. But they never solve the problem. They just teach our brain that a thought is dangerous, that we did a good thing by reacting, and that we should react again next time. It's like scratching an itch that keeps getting itchier every time you scratch it.

The real power comes from doing the opposite: allowing the thought or feeling to be there without reacting to it. We'll talk more about the tools to help you stop reacting in part 3.

But What If I Have Done These Things?

"But what if my thoughts are based on something real?"

If you've thought this, I want you to know that OCD doesn't need a perfect backstory to latch on. Even if you've made a mistake in the past—even if your thoughts feel "close to home"—you can still be stuck in the OCD cycle. And that means you can still apply these tools.

Here's the reality: People aren't perfect. We all do things we wish we could change. It's okay if you've made mistakes—every human has. OCD will try to take those past events and magnify them, distort them, and make you feel like you're defined by them.

But you're not.

Choosing to let go of guilt and shame from the past is a powerful first step toward healing. It's not about denying what happened; it's about refusing to let OCD weaponize it against you. OCD doesn't care about facts. It cares about fear. And it *lives* off your compulsions.

Mindset Reminder

No More Half-In, Half-Out

OCD won't fade because you ignore it or "wait it out." Recovery begins when you stop hoping and start practicing. Be willing to do the work—even when it's uncomfortable.

But What About Positive Mantras?

Here's a tricky one that catches a lot of us off guard: "Isn't it good to tell myself I'm okay? Aren't positive affirmations helpful?"

They can be, but with OCD, intention is everything.

Let's say a scary thought hits and you repeat a mantra like "I'm a good person. I know I'd never do that." That's not practicing acceptance—you're doing a mental compulsion that argues with the OCD. You're trying to cancel out the thought. You're trying to feel good, certain, or reassured from the thought. You're trying to fix a problem that doesn't actually exist.

That's exactly what OCD wants.

Even if it looks healthy on the surface, the behavior is feeding the cycle underneath.

But this doesn't mean you have to stay silent or let OCD steamroll you. In part 3 of this book, you'll learn the four core responses, which are new ways of talking to OCD that help create space, drop resistance, and train your brain to respond differently.

Compulsions Are What Keep OCD Alive

Intrusive thoughts are normal. We all have weird, disturbing, random thoughts sometimes. OCD becomes a disorder when we respond to those thoughts with rituals. Every time we do a compulsion—checking, avoiding, seeking reassurance, Googling, reviewing, scanning our feelings, or trying to "figure it out"—we get a hit of relief. And that relief teaches our brain the wrong lesson: *"Good job. That thought was dangerous. Do that ritual again next time."* Over time, that's what strengthens the cycle and keeps OCD going.

This is why I often say that if we pull the "C" out of OCD—if we stop compulsing—the disorder starts to fade. Strict ERP principles (which we'll discuss soon) are built on this idea through something called **ritual prevention**, which simply means not doing the behaviors that bring us relief when we're afraid of the thoughts we're having. That's how we starve OCD and take our power back.

<hr>

Key Takeaway

Compulsions are the behaviors that keep OCD alive. They feel safe, but they feed the fear. Identifying your compulsions is the first step to taking your power back. We'll talk more about the OCD cycle in the next chapter.

<hr>

Take the Next Step with OCD Space

Learning about OCD is powerful, but recovery happens when you stop responding with compulsions in the moments the urge shows up.

OCD Space is a digital recovery platform where you can work with Oscar, our clinically trained AI OCD coach, 24/7. Oscar can help you identify sneaky compulsions and practice ritual prevention in real time, so you can stop feeding OCD and keep making progress anytime, anywhere.

Join OCDspace.com and start working with Oscar today

8

THE OCD CYCLE

By now, you've learned that OCD isn't about the *content* of our thoughts; it's about how our brain reacts to uncertainty, fear, and discomfort. There's one more piece we need to understand if we're going to start breaking free: OCD operates in a predictable cycle. Until we interrupt that cycle, OCD will keep running the show.

Understanding this loop is a game changer. It's what helped me go from constantly questioning my thoughts to saying, "Oh hey, OCD—I see what you're trying to do."

Let's break it down.

Mindset Reminder

What Now?

This is where recovery begins. We stop hoping OCD will go away and start responding differently—even with uncertainty and discomfort. Trust the process. Keep practicing.

The OCD Cycle

At its core, here's how the OCD cycle works.

Step 1: Intrusive Thought (Obsession)

Something pops into our mind—an unwanted thought, image, memory, sensation, or urge. We didn't ask for it. We didn't plan it. But it's here, and it feels threatening.

Step 2: Interpretation (Meaning)

Next, we assign meaning to the thought:

- "This must mean I'm a bad person."
- "If I'm thinking this, I must want it to happen."
- "This thought can't be random—what if it's true?"
- "This thought is horrible. I just want it to go away."

Step 3: Anxiety or Distress

Our body reacts with a racing heart and mind. Dread, guilt, shame, and fear come rushing in. It feels like an emergency.

Step 4: The Desire to Remove (the Urge to Do Something)

We feel an overwhelming urge to make the thought or feeling go away. The brain starts looking for something—anything—to relieve the anxiety or find certainty.

Step 5: Compulsion (Mental or Physical)

We take an action, mental or physical, to try to get rid of the feeling and thought. This could be a ritual, a Google search, seeking reassurance, mentally reviewing, avoiding the trigger, or checking.

Step 6: Temporary Relief and Reinforcement

The anxiety fades—for now. But our brain just learned this: "Phew. That compulsion worked. Let's do that again next time."

And the cycle starts all over again.

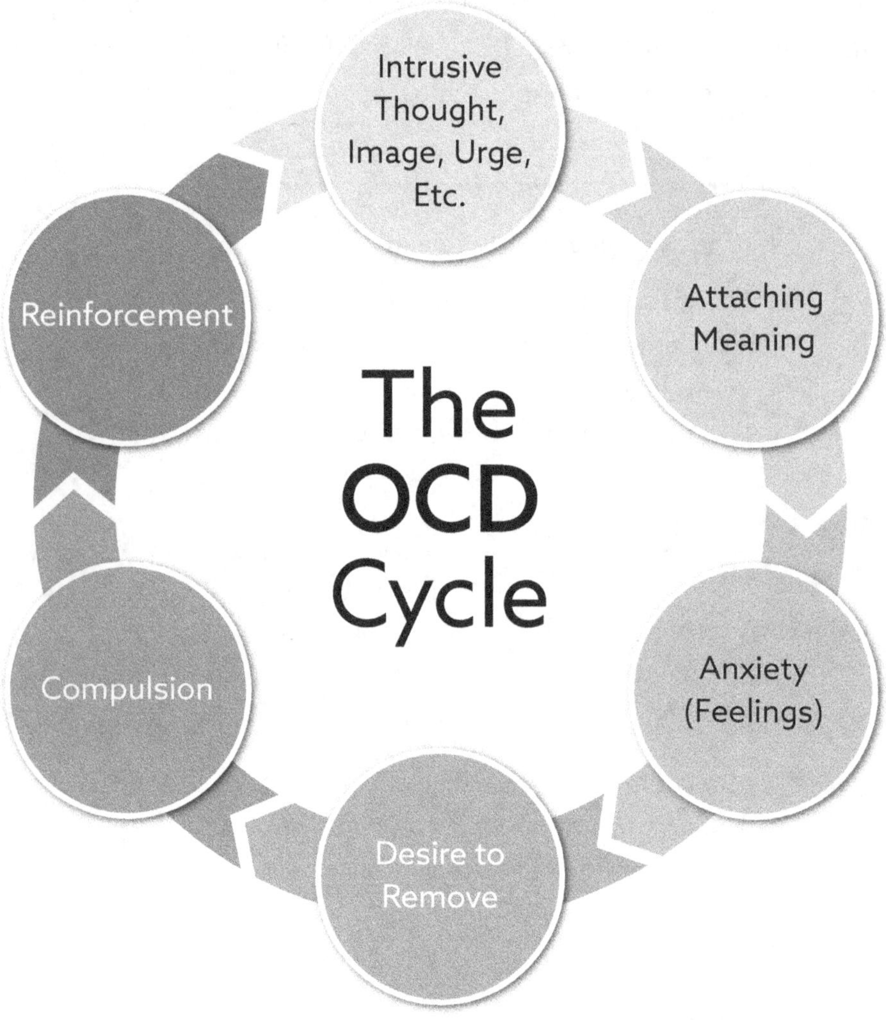

Example #1:
How Someone Moves Through the OCD Cycle

Let's say OCD sends us this intrusive thought: "What if I hit someone with my car and didn't notice?" Here's what might happen.

1. **Obsession:** This thought pops into our head after driving through a crowded street.

2. **Interpretation:** We think, "That must mean I actually could've hit someone and blocked it out." We interpret the thought as negative and potentially valid.

3. **Anxiety or distress:** We feel panic, guilt, and a tightness in our chest. Our heart starts pounding. Our brain screams, "Fix this!"

4. **Desire to remove:** We feel the overwhelming need to do something—anything—to get rid of the fear. Our mind starts racing. "Maybe if I go back and check, I'll feel better because I'll have an answer."

5. **Compulsion:** We turn the car around and retrace the entire route to check for signs of an accident.

6. **Relief and reinforcement:** We don't see anyone hurt. The anxiety fades. For a moment, we feel calm again. But our brain just learned something: "That compulsion worked. Let's use it again next time." The next time you drive, the same fear returns, only stronger.

Example #2:
Relationship OCD (ROCD)

Let's say OCD sends us this intrusive thought: "What if I don't actually love my partner?" Here's what might happen.

1. **Obsession:** The thought randomly pops into your mind while you're watching a movie together: You think, "Do I actually love them? What if I'm leading them on?"

2. **Interpretation:** You think, "If I'm questioning it, that must mean I don't really love them. I might be wasting their time, or worse, lying to both of us."

3. **Anxiety or distress:** You feel a pit in your stomach, guilt rising in your chest, maybe even nausea. The thought feels urgent and deeply unsettling.

4. **Desire to remove:** You feel the need to check—to prove to yourself that the relationship is real. "I'll just analyze how I felt this morning, how I looked at them yesterday."

5. **Compulsion:** You mentally review past moments for signs of "real" love. You compare your current relationship to past ones. You might even ask your partner, "Do you think we're really good together?"

6. **Relief and reinforcement:** Maybe you find a moment of clarity or your partner says something reassuring. You feel a wave of temporary relief. But now your brain thinks this: "That worked. Let's start this loop again tomorrow—just in case."

Example #3:
Scrupulosity/Moral OCD

Let's say OCD sends us this intrusive thought: "What if I offended God and didn't realize it?" Here's what might happen.

1. **Obsession:** After a conversation ends, you suddenly get hit with a thought: "What if I just said something sinful or offensive?"

2. **Interpretation:** You think, "If I said something wrong and don't confess or apologize, I could be punished—or I might be a bad person."

3. **Anxiety or distress:** You feel ashamed, panicked, and afraid of divine consequences or moral failure.

4. **Desire to remove:** You think, "I need to pray, confess, or apologize just to be safe." You can't relax until you "make it right."

5. **Compulsion:** You repeat a specific prayer in your head for forgiveness. You replay the conversation in your mind, trying to remember exactly what you said. You might even confess to someone close to you.

6. **Relief and reinforcement:** The anxiety fades after praying or confessing. You feel calm temporarily. But your brain logs it as this: "That is how we fix moral danger. Keep doing this." And so, the cycle continues.

Example #4:
Sexual Orientation OCD (SO-OCD)

Let's say OCD sends us this intrusive thought: "What if I'm actually gay and just in denial?" (Note: This can go in any direction and affects people of all orientations—the theme is fear, not curiosity.) Here's what might happen.

1. **Obsession:** You're scrolling through social media and see a photo of someone of your gender. Suddenly, your brain says, "Wait. Did I just find them attractive? What if I'm actually gay and have been lying to myself?"

2. **Interpretation:** You think, "If I'm having this thought, it must mean something. What if my whole identity has been fake? What if I'm living a lie?"

3. **Anxiety or distress:** Your chest tightens. Panic floods in. You feel disoriented, ashamed, and disconnected from yourself. You start mentally spiraling.

4. **Desire to remove:** You feel desperate to get rid of the doubt. "I need to prove that I'm straight" or "I need to be 100 percent sure of my orientation."

5. **Compulsion:** You scan your body for arousal. You mentally replay past sexual experiences. You compare how you feel around people of different genders. You Google orientation labels or check Reddit threads for stories like yours.

6. **Relief and reinforcement:** Maybe you feel relief after convincing yourself you're straight—or after *not* feeling aroused. But your brain learned this: "That fear was important. Next time, analyze it again." And the cycle continues.

Example #5:
Health OCD

Let's say OCD sends us this intrusive thought: "What if this headache means I have a brain tumor?" Here's what might happen.

1. **Obsession:** You wake up with a dull headache. OCD immediately jumps in: "This could be something serious. What if it's a brain tumor?"

2. **Interpretation:** You think, "Other people ignore this kind of pain, but I can't. What if I'm missing something life-threatening?"

3. **Anxiety or distress:** Your mind races. Your body tightens. You might even feel the headache more intensely because you're focused on it with anxious energy.

4. **Desire to remove:** You feel a strong pull to investigate, confirm, or eliminate the fear. "I should just check one more time. Just to be safe."

5. **Compulsion:** You start Googling brain tumor symptoms. You compare your experience to medical websites. You may ask a friend or partner, "Do you think this is serious?" Or you might check your pupils, pulse, or balance to "test" yourself.

6. **Relief and reinforcement:** Maybe you find something reassuring, or a loved one calms you down. You feel okay for a while. But your brain learned this: "We survived because we checked. Let's keep doing that." And the loop gets tighter next time.

Example #6:
Self-Harm OCD

Let's say OCD sends us this intrusive thought: "What if I snap and hurt myself?" Here's what might happen.

1. **Obsession:** You're holding a kitchen knife while cooking, and suddenly the thought hits: "What if I just stabbed myself right now?"

2. **Interpretation:** You think, "Why would I even think that? Does this mean I want to do it? Am I suicidal and don't realize it?" You start questioning your safety—and your sanity.

3. **Anxiety or distress:** Your heart races, and you feel terrified, ashamed, and overwhelmed by guilt. You might even avoid eye contact with others, worrying they'll somehow know what you're thinking.

4. **Desire to remove:** The thought feels too scary to ignore. You think, "I need to make sure I won't do anything." There's a desperate need to feel safe again.

5. **Compulsion:** You hide or throw away sharp objects. You avoid the kitchen entirely. You mentally review your past thoughts or feelings: "Have I ever wanted to hurt myself before?" You might also ask someone, "You don't think I would ever do something like that, right?"

6. **Relief and reinforcement:** Once the knife is hidden or someone reassures you, you feel a wave of relief. But your brain just learned this: "That thought was dangerous. Avoiding or checking was the right call." OCD adds another layer to the loop, and the fear comes back stronger next time.

Example #7:
Contamination OCD

Let's say OCD sends us this intrusive thought: "What if I got sick from touching that?" Here's what might happen.

1. **Obsession:** You brush up against a door handle in a public bathroom and immediately think, "What if I just picked up a dangerous virus?"

2. **Interpretation:** You think, "If I don't wash my hands thoroughly, I could get sick. Or worse, I could spread it to someone I love."

3. **Anxiety or distress:** You feel an intense wave of disgust and fear. Your skin starts to crawl. You can almost feel the germs spreading.

4. **Desire to remove:** Your brain screams, "You need to clean this off. You have to be responsible. You can't take the chance."

5. **Compulsion:** You wash your hands over and over. You may change your clothes, sanitize your phone, or avoid touching anything until you "feel clean."

6. **Relief and reinforcement:** The anxiety fades. You feel better, but your brain just learned this: "Washing made the fear go away. Let's keep doing that." And the next trigger hits even faster.

Example #8:
Existential OCD

Let's say OCD sends us this intrusive thought: "What if nothing is real?" Here's what might happen.

1. **Obsession:** You're lying in bed and the thought randomly pops in: "What if life is just a simulation? What if none of this is real?"

2. **Interpretation:** You think, "If I can't prove reality is real, how can I trust anything? What if this thought means I'm losing my mind?"

3. **Anxiety or distress:** Your stomach drops. You feel disconnected from your surroundings as you spiral into panic. You start to question your own existence.

4. **Desire to remove:** You feel desperate to "figure it out" or find proof that the world is real. You think, "I can't relax until I know for sure."

5. **Compulsion:** You Google philosophical theories. You ask friends, "Do you ever question if this is all real?" You mentally analyze past memories or physical sensations to "prove" your reality.

6. **Relief and reinforcement:** You find something that calms you down, until the thought pops up again. And now your brain thinks this: "Great job—figuring it out worked. Keep doing that next time." And the loop continues.

Example #9:
Pedophilia OCD (POCD)

Let's say OCD sends us this intrusive thought: "What if I'm attracted to children and just don't know it?" Here's what might happen.

1. **Obsession:** You see a child in public and suddenly think, "Was I just aroused? Why did I look? What does that mean?"

2. **Interpretation:** You panic. "If I'm even questioning this, I must be a predator. What if I've been hiding this from myself?"

3. **Anxiety or distress:** You feel terrified, sick to your stomach, ashamed, and disgusted. It feels like your entire identity is crumbling.

4. **Desire to remove:** You feel an urgent need to prove that you're not dangerous. "I have to know I would never act on these thoughts."

5. **Compulsion:** You avoid places where children are present. You mentally review your reaction over and over. You check your groin area for sensations. You Google stories of people with similar fears. You might even confess to someone in a desperate attempt to feel morally clean.

6. **Relief and reinforcement:** You feel slightly better after checking, avoiding, and getting reassurance. But your brain just logged that pattern as the solution: "That worked. We're safe now. Let's stay alert for the next time."

These examples demonstrate one thing clearly: The content may change, but the cycle is always the same predictable loop. That means our tools can work across any subtype.

The Recovery Response at Each Step

The empowering news is that we can interrupt the OCD cycle at any point, and the tools you're learning in this book are designed to help you do just that.

Here's how we can respond at each stage of the cycle.

Step 1: Intrusive Thought (Obsession)

Mindset: Expect and Accept. We live with OCD, which means we can expect intrusive thoughts to show up from time to time. It doesn't mean we're broken; it just means our brain is doing what it's wired to do. Think, "This is just my brain doing what it does. I expected this. I accept it."

Step 2: Interpretation (Meaning)

Tool: The Four Core Responses. This is where OCD tries to hook us with meaning. Instead of taking the bait, we respond with one of these:

- **Acceptance:** "It's okay that this thought is here. It can be here as long as it wants."
- **Uncertainty:** "Maybe it's true, maybe it's not. I'll never know for sure and that's okay."
- **Indifference:** "This thought is here. Oh, well. It is what it is."
- **Agreement:** "Yep, maybe I am a terrible person. Oh well." (This is said with sarcasm.)

These are not affirmations; they're ways of responding without feeding OCD.

Step 3: Anxiety or Distress

Tool: The Letting Go Technique. Instead of running from the feeling, we sit with it. We let it rise, peak, and pass. We don't resist it; instead, we allow it to be there without trying to get rid of it. "This feeling is temporary. I can handle it. Could I allow it to be here?"

Step 4: The Desire to Remove (the Urge to Do Something)

Mindset: Pause and Notice. Before we rush into a compulsion, we take a breath and notice the urge. That moment of awareness creates a window to choose differently. "I'm feeling the urge to do something, but that doesn't mean I have to act on it."

Step 5: Compulsion (Mental or Physical)

Tool: ERP (Exposure and Response Prevention). This is where we disrupt the pattern. We don't give in to the compulsion. We lean in, let the fear spike, and show our brain that it's okay if we don't react. "This exposure is an opportunity to teach my brain a new behavior. I'm not going to compulse. Instead, I will feel the feeling underneath the thoughts and give it permission to be here."

Step 6: Temporary Relief and Reinforcement

Mindset: Trust the Process. Maybe we feel relief, maybe we don't. It doesn't matter. The win is in how we responded. We're teaching our brain that we're in charge now, not OCD. "Whether I feel better or not, I did the hard thing. That's a win."

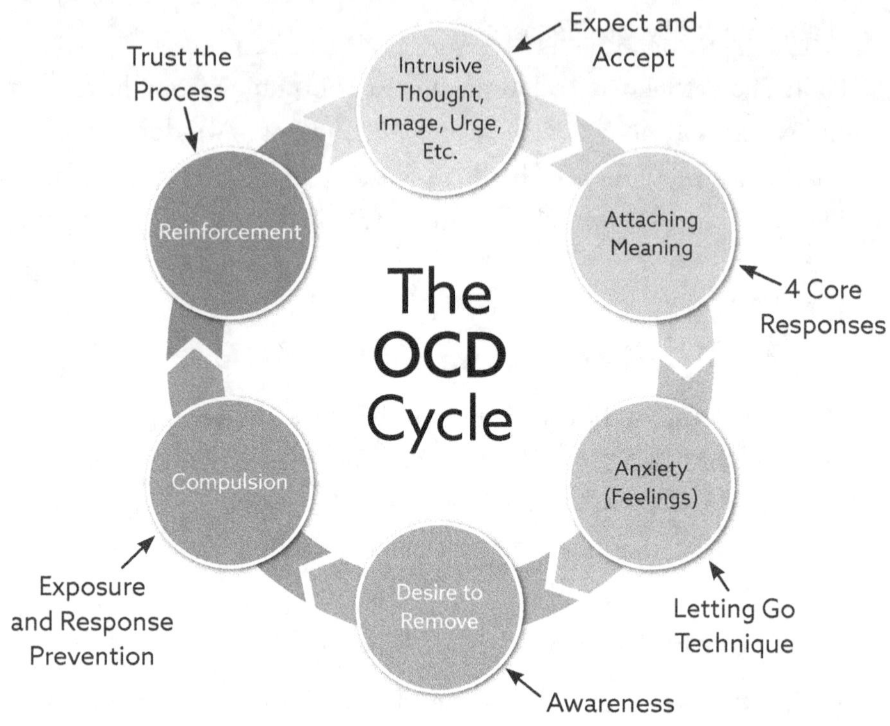

A Common Mistake That Keeps Us Stuck

If you're like most of us with OCD, you've probably had this thought: "I'll finally be free when I never have another intrusive thought or feeling again."

Here's the tough truth: Recovery isn't about getting rid of the thoughts. It's about teaching our brain not to care if or when they happen.

When we make the absence of intrusive thoughts our goal, we unintentionally send the message to our brain that those thoughts are dangerous, that they must go away permanently for us to feel safe or happy. This keeps the OCD cycle alive because we're labeling the thoughts negatively.

When we shift our focus to no longer reacting to the thoughts, everything changes. Our new goal becomes "I can have any thought and still live the life I want."

That's freedom, and that's where we're headed next with the skills you'll learn throughout this book.

Pro Tip: Watch Your Language—Literally

Remember earlier in the book when we talked about not labeling thoughts as *weird*, *disgusting*, or *horrible*?

That wasn't just about tone—it's about neuroscience.

When we use emotionally charged language to describe a thought, our brain's fear center (the amygdala) picks up on that and flags the thought as dangerous. The more we call a thought *horrible*, the more our brain believes it is.

Instead, try shifting to neutral or observational language like "That was an interesting thought," "That's a sticky one today," or "OCD's being chatty again."

This might feel silly at first, but it's a subtle and powerful way to teach your brain that the thought isn't a threat—it's just noise.

Key Takeaway

The OCD cycle keeps us stuck when we react the way OCD wants us to. When we shift our mindset and apply the right tools, we take back control one step at a time.

Take the Next Step with OCD Space

Understanding the OCD cycle is an important important first step. But when you're stuck in it, things can get confusing fast, especially in the moment.

That's exactly why I built OCD Space and Oscar, the world's first clinically trained AI OCD coach. Oscar is designed to help you understand how you're getting pulled into the cycle and guide you through responding differently, in real time.

**Start your free trial at
OCDspace.com**

9

WHEN OCD USES OUR BODY AGAINST US

Our symptoms aren't proof of danger; they're OCD trying to get our attention.

Since we live with OCD, we know this feeling: Our thoughts flood in, and then our body responds hard. Our heart races. We feel dizzy, sick, or lightheaded. Our stomach drops. We might even feel like we're leaving our body, like we're watching our life happen from the outside. This is anxiety doing what anxiety does. It's the fight-or-flight system firing off, convinced that something is wrong.

This is where it can get tricky—because OCD sees those symptoms as leverage.

"See? This Means Something's Wrong"

OCD doesn't just use our thoughts against us, it uses the body too:

- "You're dizzy? That means you're about to pass out."
- "You feel detached? That proves you're losing control."

- "Your chest is tight? That's because you did something wrong."

OCD hijacks our physical sensations and spins a story. This makes the thoughts feel true. The reality is that these symptoms are likely not evidence of danger, just our nervous system responding to a thought because of the meaning we've attached to it.

Mindset Reminder

Discomfort Isn't Danger

When OCD triggers anxiety in your body, it will feel urgent and real. But you don't need certainty to move forward. Embrace uncertainty. Tolerate discomfort. Keep living anyway.

How Physical Symptoms Fit into the OCD Cycle

Sometimes OCD leads with a thought, but other times it leads with a sensation. Either way, the cycle is the same. Let's tie this back to the OCD cycle you just learned about:

1. **A physical sensation hits** (anxiety, adrenaline, tight chest, dizziness, "off" feeling, etc.).
2. We assign meaning to it. ("What if this means something is wrong with me?")
3. **Our nervous system reacts even more** with fear and urgency.
4. OCD uses those symptoms to convince us the threat is real.
5. We do a compulsion, often to get rid of the *feeling*, not just the thought.
6. We feel temporary relief, but we reinforce the wrong message for our brain.

It's not just "What if I hit someone with my car?" It becomes "I feel dizzy and disoriented, which means I was distracted while driving. Maybe I hit someone. I need to go check. Okay, I've checked, and feel better. This was the right thing to do, and I'll do it again next time."

See how sneaky that is?

Common Physical Symptoms of Anxiety That OCD Might Hijack

- Vertigo or lightheadedness (feeling dizzy)
- Nausea or stomach cramps
- Tightness in chest
- Derealization (feeling detached from your surroundings)
- Depersonalization (feeling detached from yourself)
- Racing heart
- Tingling or numbness
- Tension or shaking
- Panic attacks

These are normal symptoms of anxiety. They can feel overwhelming, but they're not dangerous. Most importantly, they are not proof that your intrusive thought is true.

Example #1: Vertigo as "Evidence"

Let's say your OCD focuses on health, driving, or losing control. You feel a wave of vertigo hit you out of nowhere. OCD immediately jumps in:

- "This means something is seriously wrong."
- "You're about to pass out. Do something!"
- "This proves you hit someone and blocked it out."

Now your fear response gets even stronger. You do a compulsion by checking your body, retracing your steps, or Googling your symptoms. And the OCD cycle keeps spinning.

Here's what's actually happening and what OCD doesn't want you to see: You felt dizzy because you were anxious, not because you were about to faint or did something wrong.

Example #2: Racing Heart or Tingling as "Heart Attack Proof"

I had a coaching client who noticed his heart racing and his arms tingling. Here's what OCD told him:

- "This is it. You're having a heart attack."
- "You need to go to the ER."
- "This proves something's seriously wrong with your body."

In reality, these were textbook symptoms of anxiety and panic. So here's what we practiced saying: "This is just anxiety. Maybe it's a heart attack, maybe it's not. I'm not solving this today. I'm allowed to feel discomfort without turning it into an emergency."

Important Note

If you're ever experiencing new or unusual physical symptoms—especially ones that are intense, persistent, or feel medically concerning—it's always a good idea to consult with a licensed medical professional.

There's a difference between genuine health advocacy and compulsive checking.

Once your doctor has cleared you, OCD may try to convince you to keep questioning it. That's when we need to recognize OCD's voice and practice letting go of the urge to solve.

What to Do Instead

When anxiety symptoms show up, try this:

1. **Name what's happening:** "This is anxiety in my body. I expected this, and I accept its presence."
2. **Let it be there without reacting:** "These symptoms are uncomfortable, but they're allowed to be here."
3. **Use the four core responses:** acceptance, uncertainty, indifference, agreement. More on this is part 3.
4. **Let go of the need to fix it:** "I don't need to feel better right now. I just need to let it pass on its own time."

Key Takeaway

The physical symptoms of anxiety are not proof of danger. OCD will try to use normal symptoms of anxiety against us to get our attention and make us compulse.

We get to choose how we respond, and that response is what rewires our brain.

10

THE LIES OCD TELLS US

OCD lies to us to keep us stuck in the cycle. It disguises itself as *logic*, *morality*, *safety*, or even *love*. If we're not aware of its tricks, we'll keep falling for them over and over again.

Let me be clear: OCD doesn't care about the truth. It cares about control and perceived safety. The more we try to reason with it, prove it wrong, or make it go away, the stronger OCD gets.

In this chapter, we're going to call out some of OCD's most common lies and replace them with truth. Once we know the game OCD tries to play, we can stop playing it.

Lie #1: "I don't really have OCD."

This is one of the most common lies OCD uses when we're starting to get better. The doubt creeps in: "What if I've just been using OCD as an excuse? What if this is actually real and I've been avoiding it?"

Here's what's wild: Doubting our diagnosis is actually a symptom of OCD. OCD loves to make us question the one thing that gives us relief because if we don't believe it's OCD, we'll go right back to compulsing.

Truth: OCD makes us question everything, including whether we even have OCD. That's how it keeps its grip. Keep using the tools anyway.

Lie #2: "This time is different."

You've been down this road before. You've had intrusive thoughts, done exposures, resisted compulsions—and now a new theme shows up. Suddenly, OCD says, "This thought feels different. This isn't like the other ones."

This lie works because OCD is a shapeshifter. I call this the OCD Ninja because OCD will sneak up on us in an attempt to find a topic that gets our attention.

The themes may change, but the process of recovery is always the same.

Truth: It's the same cycle, just wearing a different costume. We treat it the same way every time.

Lie #3: "You're the exception."

OCD loves to isolate us. It tells us lies like these:

- "Other people can recover, but you're different."
- "If they knew your thoughts, they'd be disgusted."
- "Maybe other people have bad thoughts, but yours are the worst!"
- "This isn't even OCD, it's just who you are."

Truth: You're not the exception. You're just like every single person with OCD. Every person I've ever coached has felt like they were the one person who couldn't be helped or whose thoughts were the worst (even compared to other OCDers). Every one of them started to heal when they stopped believing this lie. If you're new to OCD recovery, I bet reading this just now triggered doubt that this book will even help you. That's proof that OCD will do anything it can to get us to stop doing the work.

Lie #4: "If I'm thinking it, it must mean something."

OCD's favorite move is to confuse thoughts with truth. It'll say things like these:

- "You wouldn't be thinking that if it wasn't important."
- "If you didn't want it, you wouldn't be obsessing over it."
- "Normal people don't think this way."

Truth: Intrusive thoughts are meaningless mental noise, or what I like to call junk content. Everyone has them. The difference is that those of us with OCD react to them, and that's what keeps them around.

Lie #5: "OCD can switch subtypes and I should fear that."

OCD tells us, "Since OCD changes themes, you can't trust yourself. You'll always have something to obsess about. So what's the point?"

But here's the reframe: Yes, OCD can morph, but that means our recovery tools work across the board. Once we stop buying into the fear and start focusing on how we respond, we gain real traction.

Truth: Subtypes may shift, but the cycle stays the same, and that means we can learn how to handle it consistently.

Lie #6: "This feels so real."

Yup. It does, and that's what makes OCD sticky. The anxiety, the guilt, and bodily sensations all *feel* real in the body, so we assume they must be true.

But fear is a feeling, not a fact. Just because something feels intense doesn't mean it's meaningful.

Truth: OCD mimics real emotion to get our attention, but it's just a false alarm.

Lie #7: "Just do the compulsion this one last time."

This is OCD's most manipulative lie, and also the most believable. It makes the fear feel so real, so urgent, so unbearable that we think things like these:

- "Okay, I'll just check this one time. I'll have an answer, and then I'll stop."
- "I'll confess one more thing. Just to be safe."
- "I'll do the exposure tomorrow. I just need a break today."

Truth: There is no last time. Every compulsion reinforces the cycle and feeds the OCD more. The only way out is through, which means leaning into the discomfort and choosing to break the pattern right now.

Lie #8: "I'm a horrible person for thinking these thoughts."

This is OCD's go-to guilt trip. It convinces us that the *thought* equals the *person*, and that if we were really good, we wouldn't even be capable of thinking such things.

As we discussed earlier, everyone has strange, intrusive, even disturbing thoughts. What makes OCD different is that we care. We don't want these thoughts. We react to them because they go against our deepest values.

Truth: The more we believe we're "horrible people" for thinking certain thoughts, the longer OCD keeps us stuck in the cycle. Letting go of the guilt and shame toward these thoughts can become a pathway to freedom from this lie OCD tells us.

Lie #9: "OCD recovery is confusing. I don't know how to do it."

This lie hits when we're overwhelmed, exhausted, and discouraged. OCD wants us to believe we're too broken, too far gone, or just not "getting it."

But recovery isn't about doing everything perfectly. It's about showing up with whatever energy we have in that moment, using our tools, and taking small steps even when we don't feel ready.

Truth: You're learning as you go. It's okay if you don't have it all figured out yet. None of us did at the start.

Lie #10: "This time I'll get an answer, and it will stick."

Ah, the false promise of certainty. OCD dangles this lie like bait: "Just do this one more compulsion. One more Google search. One more deep mental review. Then you'll finally have peace."

That peace never lasts. OCD doesn't want an answer—it wants 100 percent certainty, 100 percent of the time. This can't be achieved.

Truth: Certainty is a trap. Peace doesn't come from solving. It comes from letting go of needing to have an answer 100 percent of the time.

Lie #11: "I've been living a lie."

This lie attacks our identity. It shows up in SO-OCD, ROCD, real event OCD, POCD—any theme where OCD says, "You haven't been honest with yourself. You've faked your entire life." It feels like a collapse of everything we know about ourselves. But again, that fear is the evidence of OCD at work.

Truth: OCD isn't revealing some hidden truth; he's exploiting your deepest values and fears.

Lie #12: "I'm back at square one. It's like all my work was for nothing."

Setbacks are a normal part of recovery. When they happen, OCD loves to swoop in and say, "See? You're not making progress. You're stuck. You'll never get better."

That's not true.

Every exposure you've done and every urge you've resisted is part of your healing. There's no such thing as a setback because at any given moment we can choose to use our tools, which help us step out of the OCD cycle.

Truth: You're not back at square one. You're one decision away from showing OCD that you're in charge by utilizing your tools.

Key Takeaway

OCD's power comes from lies. First, we build awareness. Then, we choose to stop believing the lies OCD tells us. That's how we start to reclaim our power and our lives.

11

COMMON COGNITIVE DISTORTIONS

OCD's favorite hobby is twisting the truth until it feels like a fact. It doesn't just send us scary thoughts—it distorts reality. It takes a single idea, a random spike, a fleeting doubt, and turns it into an emergency.

This is where *cognitive distortions* come in.

Cognitive distortions are mental habits that exaggerate fear, shrink perspective, and fuel compulsions. They're not exclusive to OCD, but OCD absolutely thrives on them. The more we buy into these distortions, the more we reinforce the idea that our thoughts are dangerous.

The good news is that once we recognize these patterns, we can start to interrupt them.

We can say, "Wait a second—that's OCD talking. Not me."

Let's break down some of the most common distortions that keep us stuck.

1. Black-and-White Thinking

The distortion: "If I'm not 100 percent certain, I must be totally unsure," or "If I had one weird thought, I must be a monster."

This is also known as all-or-nothing thinking. It's a distortion that turns everything into extremes. There's no middle ground. We're either safe or doomed. Good or evil. Guilty or innocent. OCD loves this one because it makes any gray area feel intolerable.

2. Thought-Action Fusion

The distortion: "If I think it, I might do it" or "If I thought it, it's basically the same as it happening."

This one's huge for OCD. OCD tells us that just having a thought is morally or physically dangerous. That it increases the chance that something bad will happen. That it *means* something about us.

OCD might tell us that thinking something is equivalent to doing it—or that it means there should be consequences.

Here's the truth: A thought is just a thought. It has no power until we give it attention. Whether it's harm OCD, intrusive sexual thoughts, or blasphemous spikes, thinking it doesn't make it real.

3. Emotional Reasoning

The distortion: "Because I feel anxious, something must be wrong."

OCD hijacks our feelings and uses them as evidence. If we feel guilty, it must mean we did something wrong. If we feel anxious, it must mean there's danger. If we feel uncertain, it must mean we're in denial.

This distortion trains us to trust our fear instead of our values.

4. Catastrophizing

The distortion: "If I don't figure this out, something terrible will happen."

OCD loves to escalate things. It doesn't say, "Maybe you made a mistake." It says, "If you don't solve this *right now*, your life will fall apart."

This distortion turns mild uncertainty into worst-case scenarios. It fuels compulsions out of panic.

5. Magical Thinking

The distortion: "If I think or do this, I'll cause something to happen."

This is common in contamination OCD, religious OCD, and superstitious themes. "If I don't wash perfectly, someone might die," or "If I don't pray a certain way, I'm inviting evil," or "If I don't confess, I might go to hell."

It makes us believe that our thoughts or behaviors have more power than they actually do.

6. Mental Filtering

The distortion: We only notice what seems to confirm our fear. We overlook the 99 percent of life that's safe, good, or fine, and we obsess over the 1 percent that feels threatening. "What if that look from my friend meant I offended them?" or "What if I enjoyed that thought for a second?" or "What if that one article online means it's all true?"

OCD is a master at filtering out evidence that contradicts his story.

7. Mind Reading

The distortion: "I know what others are thinking, and it's bad."

This distortion shows up in relationship OCD, social anxiety, and scrupulosity. "They think I'm a terrible person," or "They're offended, and I have to fix it," or "Everyone saw me mess up, I know it."

Here's the reality: We're terrible at reading minds.

Constantly trying to guess other people's thoughts fuels reassurance-seeking, apologizing, confessing, and avoiding.

8. Labeling

The distortion: "I'm a fraud. I'm disgusting. I'm broken."

This distortion collapses our entire identity into a single thought or behavior. It's the difference between "I had a weird thought" and "I *am* a horrible person."

OCD uses this to fuel shame, and the more shame we feel, the more we engage in compulsions to try to fix ourselves.

When It Becomes About Morality and Responsibility

For many of us with OCD, the fear isn't just about what might happen; it's about what it might say about who we are.

This is where OCD goes beyond anxiety and becomes a moral threat. OCD tells us things like these:

- "Only a terrible person would think that."
- "You have to figure this out or you're being irresponsible."
- "You owe it to the world to make sure nothing bad ever happens."

This is called hyper-responsibility, and it's a major driver of compulsions. It's also deeply tied to the need to be good, do good, and feel good all the time, which, of course, no one can realistically achieve. Many of the distortions you've just read about are fueled by this internal need to prove that you're morally good.

Here's the truth: Thoughts aren't moral. Feelings aren't moral. Being a good person has nothing to do with the content of our OCD. We don't have to fix, prove, or purify every mental experience. We just have to learn how to see it for what it is: OCD doing his thing again, trying to pull us into the OCD cycle.

When we stop believing it, everything changes.

What About Manifestation?

I hear this one all the time from people in the OCD community: "What if I'm manifesting my fears just by thinking about them?"

OCD loves this one. It sounds spiritual, profound, even empowering, but under the surface, it's just another fear dressed up in disguise.

Let's break it down.

Manifestation Is About Intent + Action

Manifestation typically refers to focusing on something we want and aligning our actions and energy to help make it a reality.

Let's say I sit on my couch and think, "I want a million dollars to show up in my mailbox."

I can think that thought as many times as I want. Unless I take massive action—start a business, invest, network, build something—it's *very* unlikely to happen.

Why?

Because manifestation doesn't work by pure thought alone. It involves intentional energy, aligned effort, and usually a lot of hard work.

Now let's compare that to how OCD frames it: "I thought about harming someone. What if that means I will?" or "I imagined getting sick. What if I manifest that into reality?"

These are not desires. They're not goals. They're unwanted, fear-based thoughts. You didn't *choose* the thought. You don't *want* the outcome. You're just scared of it, and that fear is fueling the cycle.

But What If I Think I'll Throw Up and Then I Feel Sick?

This is another one I hear often: "Every time I think about throwing up, I feel nauseous. Isn't that proof I'm manifesting it?"

Not quite.

This ties back to the chapter on anxiety and bodily sensations. When we fixate on a physical symptom, we actually increase our awareness of and sensitivity to it.

If I obsess over whether my stomach feels weird, it probably will start to feel weird. Not because I manifested it but because I'm scanning my body like a hawk.

OCD is great at twisting this. It says, "See? You thought about it, and now it's happening."

In reality, you're just noticing normal physical sensations that come from anxiety.

If we stopped believing that every thought had the power to manifest reality, that fear would lose all its weight.

Final Thought

Cognitive distortions are not our fault. They're mental reflexes that come from fear, trauma, and uncertainty. Once we learn to recognize them, we can start responding differently. We can catch OCD mid-lie, pause, and say, "Thanks for your input. I'm not going to give this thought weight, but it's welcome to be here for as long as it needs to be."

We don't need to fix our thoughts; we just need to stop believing their distortions.

In the coming chapters, we'll discuss how to talk to OCD more effectively so that we don't get tangled up in the OCD cycle.

Key Takeaway

OCD's power depends on distorted thinking. The moment we recognize those distortions and choose not to believe them, we start taking our power back.

PART 3

THE FOUR CORE RESPONSES THAT CHANGE EVERYTHING

By now, you understand the OCD cycle and how it keeps us stuck.

But understanding isn't enough. Recovery happens when we learn to respond differently. Not once. Not perfectly. But over and over again over time.

The four core responses in this section are how we interrupt the cycle. They're how we teach our brain a new way to respond to uncomfortable thoughts and feelings. They help us sit in uncertainty without reacting by compulsing.

The four core responses are foundational skills of OCD recovery, and they're how we take our lives back from OCD.

Why This Matters

If we keep reacting to OCD with fear and urgency, OCD wins.

When we instead respond with acceptance, uncertainty, indifference, or agreement, we teach our brain to think, "This thought doesn't need my attention. I don't need to solve it. I'm choosing freedom."

It won't feel normal at first to respond using these skills. It might feel unnatural, wrong, irresponsible, awkward, and uncomfortable. That's because your brain has been conditioned to treat these thoughts like threats.

These four core responses are the exact tools that help rewire that fear response so the anxiety fades naturally and you stop fueling the cycle.

One important note: The four core responses aren't magic phrases that "fix" OCD on their own. They work because they help us respond differently *and then* resist the urge to do compulsions. If we say a response but still ritualize (checking, analyzing, Googling, seeking reassurance, reviewing, scanning feelings, etc.), we're still feeding OCD. The real breakthrough happens when we use these responses and then choose not to compulse. That's what rewires the brain.

What to Expect in This Section

For each of the four core responses, you'll get the following:

- A breakdown of what it is (and isn't)
- Why it works neurologically
- Real examples across subtypes
- What to do when it feels hard
- How to practice it in real life

The goal here is to have you practice using these responses when uncomfortable thoughts and feelings come up. Experiment with all of them and then pick the ones that resonate with you the most. Use those over and over again.

To this day I still use the four core responses. Why? Because they work effectively to keep me out of the OCD cycle so I can live my life the way I want to.

I want that for you too. It's time to learn and practice the skills that matter.

Take the Next Step with OCD Space

Now that you can see how OCD pulls you into the cycle, the next step is learning how to respond differently when it tries to pull you back in.

OCD Space is a digital recovery platform designed to help you practice new responses when OCD hits in real life. You can work with Oscar, our clinically trained AI OCD coach, anytime you need support.

Oscar will help you practice the four core responses in real time so you can change the meaning your brain assigns to intrusive thoughts and feelings.

Join OCDspace.com and start working with Oscar today

12

ACCEPTANCE

This thought is here . . . and
I'm letting it be here.

If you're like most of us, your first reaction to intrusive thoughts is to resist them. To fight them. To push them away, suppress them, question them, analyze them, or try to cancel them out.

That makes total sense. These thoughts feel scary and uncomfortable. They might feel unacceptable. So our instinct is to get rid of them as fast as possible.

Here's the twist though. OCD recovery is paradoxical. The harder we try to resist thoughts, the more we get stuck with them. The more we push against a thought, the more power we give it. The more we try to figure it out, the deeper we sink.

That's why the first core response in recovery is acceptance.

> ## Mindset Reminder
>
> ### Practice > Perfection
>
> You don't have to do this perfectly. OCD will try to turn recovery into another obsession. Your job is simply to practice—and embrace uncertainty as you do.

What Is Acceptance in OCD Recovery?

Acceptance sounds like this: "Maybe I'm not the biggest fan of this thought or sensation. I didn't choose it. But it's here and I'm allowing it to be here without trying to change it or get rid of it."

We're not saying the thought or sensation is good or bad. We're not necessarily liking it. We're simply accepting reality as it is, in this moment, without needing to fix, avoid, or control it.

The need to fix, avoid, or control the thought or feeling is what's getting us tangled up in it and pushing us deeper into the OCD cycle.

Why It Works

Our brains learn through experience.

When we allow a thought or sensation to be there without reacting to it—without doing a compulsion—our brain starts to think, "Hey, maybe this isn't actually dangerous. Maybe I don't need to react to it because Zach didn't."

Over time, the anxiety starts to fade on its own. Not because we made the thought go away but because we stopped treating it like a threat.

A Note on What Acceptance Feels Like at First

It's important to understand that when we *start* using accepting statements, we're not going to feel accepting right away. In fact, it might feel fake, forced, or scary.

You might say, "This thought is here, and I accept it"—but inside, your body is screaming, "Nope. I hate this. This is terrifying."

That's okay. That's normal.

Don't be surprised if you also feel skeptical. OCD might jump in and say, "I know you're just pretending to be accepting. This will never work." That's part of the process too. Don't deny those thoughts either. Don't argue with them.

Instead, respond with the very tool you're practicing: an accepting statement. "This doubt is here and that's okay. I'm letting it be here. It's okay if I feel skeptical."

Acceptance is not a feeling at first. It's a choice, followed by a behavioral decision. With repetition—day after day, thought after thought, sensation after sensation—that acceptance begins to settle in naturally. Our brain starts to believe it. Our body starts to calm down. It starts with the repetition, not the feeling.

Keep practicing, even if it doesn't feel like it's working right away. It is.

Common Objections to Acceptance

OCD will throw everything he's got at this one:

- "If I accept this thought, I'm saying it's okay."
- "If I don't fight it, I must want it."
- "What if acceptance means I give up and something bad happens?"

- "What if I accept this feeling and something bad happens?"

Remember: Acceptance is not approval. It's not giving in. It's letting go of the need to control what we can't control—the random thoughts and sensations that bubble up. You've probably already tried controlling your thoughts, and my guess is that it didn't work. This is why shifting our energy to what we can control (how we respond) is all that matters.

My Turning Point with Acceptance

When I first started struggling with intrusive thoughts—especially around SO-OCD, harm OCD, and POCD—I believed they were the worst, most unacceptable thoughts on the face of the planet.

There was a 0 percent chance I would ever "accept" them. In my mind, if I accepted the thoughts, that meant I *agreed* with them. If I agreed with them, that made me a horrible person. So I did what felt logical: I rejected them. I pushed back. I thought that rejecting the thoughts proved I wasn't "that kind of person."

What I didn't realize was that this very mindset—the need to reject, resist, and prove—was keeping me stuck in a constant state of fear, shame, and exhaustion. It led to depression and feeling like I wanted to give up.

Eventually, I hit a breaking point. I had nothing left to lose, so I tried something different: I leaned into the idea of acceptance.

What I learned changed everything:

- **Acceptance doesn't mean agreement.** It doesn't mean I want the thought, like the thought, or identify with it.
- **I must fully accept that I have OCD.** As someone with OCD, my brain is going to send me random thoughts, images, urges, and sensations that feel out of alignment with my values and who I feel I am.

- **If the thoughts are just a symptom of OCD, I don't have to assign them meaning anymore.** OCD is a medical condition, and just like a cough is a symptom of a cold, intrusive thoughts are a symptom of OCD.

When that clicked, I realized something huge: I could allow the thoughts to be there. I could stop trying to prove, analyze, or erase them. I could accept them—not as truth, not as identity—but as junk content from OCD.

"I've radically accepted that I have OCD. And that means I will have random, unwanted thoughts from time to time. They don't mean anything about who I am. They are just symptoms of the disorder."

Taking the Leap of Faith

Using tools like acceptance, uncertainty, indifference, and agreement often feels like a leap of faith.

We've spent so long believing that staying on guard keeps us safe. So when we drop the compulsions and stop fighting the thoughts, it feels risky—like something bad might happen. That leap is where freedom begins. It's how we retrain our brains not to fear the thoughts, and it's how we start to get our lives back.

How to Practice Radical Acceptance

Start with a trigger. Let's say you have this thought: "What if I cheated and don't remember?"

Here's how you respond:

1. Pause and name the thought: "Okay, there's the cheating fear again."
2. Feel the anxiety. Let it rise. Don't resist it.
3. Say to yourself, "This thought is here and it's okay. I'm allowing it to be here and pass on its own time."
4. Try your best not to engage, review, or seek reassurance.
5. To the best of your ability, bring your focus back to your day. It's okay if the thought is still there.

Every time you do this, you're showing your brain, "This isn't worth reacting to anymore. It's not worth giving it any importance."

Real Examples Across Subtypes

Harm OCD

Trigger: "What if I snap and hurt someone?"
Response: "It's okay that this thought is bubbling up. I can let it sit here without needing to prove it wrong."

Relationship OCD

Trigger: "What if I'm not really in love?"
Response: "It's okay that this thought is here. I don't need to solve it. I'll let it stay if it wants to."

POCD

Trigger: "What if I was attracted to that child?"
Response: "This thought is just a random thought. I'm not reacting. It's okay if it's here or if it passes on its own time."

Contamination OCD

Trigger: "What if this surface gave me a disease?"

Response: "Yep, my brain is firing off again. I accept that this fear is here."

Just Right OCD

Trigger: "I didn't say that perfectly. Now something bad might happen."

Response: "That's an OCD thought. I'm choosing to move on without fixing it."

Let's look at an example.

1. **Trigger/intrusive thought:** "What if I lose control and hurt someone I love?"
2. **Interpretation/meaning attached to the thought:** "This must mean I'm dangerous or broken."
3. **Recovery response option (acceptance):** "This thought is here, and that's okay. I'm not pushing it away."

Rumination: Where Acceptance Breaks Down

By now, you already know that rumination is one of OCD's most common compulsions. It's the mental ritual of analyzing, debating, reviewing, and trying to "figure it out" until we feel relief.

And this is important: Rumination is usually the exact moment acceptance breaks down. OCD doesn't just want us to feel anxious—it wants us to respond with urgency. It wants us to take the thought seriously and start solving it.

So even when we *try* to practice acceptance, OCD will often pull us right back into mental compulsions:

- "Okay, but what if it's actually true?"
- "What does this say about me?"
- "Why am I thinking this?"

- "Let me just be sure."

This might feel like we're being responsible. But what we're really doing is ritualizing.

Acceptance vs. Rumination

Acceptance sounds like:

- "Maybe, maybe not."
- "I don't need to solve this."
- "I can feel discomfort and still live my life."

Rumination sounds like:

- "Let me think about this a little longer."
- "I need to understand what this means."
- "I can't move on until I feel certain."

So here's a simple truth: You can't accept and ruminate at the same time.

Example: Intrusive Thought → Rumination → Acceptance

Let's say you're holding your baby and you get a random intrusive thought: "What if I dropped her?"

That thought hits like a punch in the stomach. And OCD immediately tries to pull you into rumination:

- "Why would I think that?"
- "Does that mean I secretly want to hurt her?"
- "What if this is a sign I'm dangerous?"
- "What if I lose control?"
- "Should I put her down just to be safe?"
- "Let me check how I feel. Do I feel anxious enough?"
- "Normal people don't think this… so what's wrong with me?"

Notice what's happening: OCD is trying to turn one intrusive thought into an *emergency investigation*.

This is where acceptance steps in. The goal isn't to prove the thought wrong—it's to stop feeding it.

An accepting response might sound like: "Maybe I could drop her. Maybe I couldn't. I'm not solving this." Or, "I'm going to hold her, feel the discomfort, and keep living."

That response is powerful because it stops the mental ritual. It pulls you out of rumination and back into reality.

The Missing Piece: Ritual Prevention

This is why acceptance isn't just a statement—it's a *behavioral choice*.

When we practice acceptance, we also practice ritual prevention, meaning we don't do the behaviors that bring relief—especially the mental ones.

Because if we say an accepting response but then spend the next thirty minutes analyzing the thought, **OCD** still wins.

How to Apply Acceptance in Real Life

Acceptance isn't saying the perfect phrase. It's making one simple decision in the moment: "I'm not solving this."

And then returning to your life, even with discomfort still in your body.

Here's a short script you can use anytime you catch yourself starting to spiral:

- "I'm going to practice feeling uncomfortable while not ritualizing."
- "Maybe it's true, maybe it's not."
- "Back to my life."
- "I had this thought, and that's okay."

At first, this will feel unfinished—like you're walking away from something important. That's normal. That's the withdrawal from the compulsion.

But every time you redirect your brain away from rumination, you're doing the deepest form of acceptance there is: you're allowing uncertainty without trying to fix it.

Key Takeaway

Acceptance means allowing the thought to be there without reacting to it. It doesn't mean you're agreeing with the thought or that you like it. It's simply about accepting its presence.

It's one of the first steps toward freedom. Accepting that we have OCD, and that a symptom of OCD is random, junk-content thoughts, gives us permission to stop assigning them meaning.

Call to Action

Practice Acceptance Statements

For the next few days, when a thought or fear pops up, try using acceptance statements like these:

- "This thought is here, and I'm allowing it to be here."
- "I may not like this feeling, but I'm willing to feel it."
- "I'm choosing to accept this moment as it is."
- "It's okay that this thought is here."
- "It's okay that (insert the feeling you're experiencing) is here."

Even if it feels forced at first, stick with it. Remember, acceptance isn't about liking the thought. It's about letting go of the fight. Let your nervous system learn that "this isn't an emergency."

13

UNCERTAINTY

What if I never get the answer?

Your reply to the question above? "Then I'll learn to live without it."

If there's one thing OCD cannot stand, it's uncertainty. It wants guarantees and definitive answers. When OCD doesn't get certainty, we are flooded with fear, shame, doubt, and guilt until we go looking for reassurance or do a compulsion to "make sure."

It's a trap. The harder we chase certainty, the further away it gets.

OCD's Addiction to Certainty

OCD thrives on questions that can't be answered with 100 percent certainty:

- "What if I hurt someone and forgot?"
- "What if I don't really love my partner?"

- "What if I secretly want the thing I'm afraid of?"
- "What if I sinned and didn't realize it?"
- "What if I got contaminated and now I'm spreading it?"
- "What if I have a life-threatening disease and the doctors missed it?"
- "What if I have a heart attack and drop dead?"

It doesn't matter how many times you answer OCD. It always follows up with "But how can you be sure?"

OCD isn't looking for the truth. It's looking for *certainty*, and certainty is something we don't get in this life.

Not about our thoughts.

Not about our relationships.

Not even about our health, our past, or our future.

This can be a tough pill to swallow for most OCDers at the beginning. It was for me.

But the freedom we experience when we make the conscious decision to let go of needing an answer with 100 percent certainty is life-changing.

The Real Shift: Choosing Uncertainty on Purpose

Recovery doesn't mean finally figuring it out. It means making peace with the fact that *we won't and that's okay.*

That might sound scary at first or even frustrating, but it's actually where freedom begins. When we stop chasing certainty, we stop fueling the cycle. We stop feeding OCD. We take back our energy and attention so we can focus on living a values-based life.

OCD will always ask, "What if this thought is true?"

You can answer, "Maybe it is, maybe it's not. I'll never know for sure and I'm okay with that."

Why Uncertainty Is So Powerful

From a brain science perspective, choosing uncertainty does two things:

1. **It removes the compulsion.** You're no longer reacting to the thought with problem-solving.
2. **It builds distress tolerance.** You teach your brain that you can survive discomfort without getting rid of it.

The more you sit in uncertainty, the more your brain learns that nothing bad has happened and it can stop sending the alarm. That's how rewiring begins.

What Living with Uncertainty Sounds Like

Let's look at how this works across different subtypes:

Harm OCD

Trigger: "What if I lose control and hurt someone?"
Response: "Maybe I will, maybe I won't. I'm not solving this."

SO-OCD

Trigger: "What if I'm gay and just don't know it?"
Response: "Could be. Could not be. I'm not chasing that answer anymore."

Scrupulosity/Moral OCD

Trigger: "What if I offended God?"
Response: "Maybe I did. I'll never be sure. That's okay."

Contamination OCD

Trigger: "What if this surface had something dangerous on it?"
Response: "Maybe it did. I'm choosing to move forward anyway."

Just Right OCD

Trigger: "What if I didn't say that perfectly?"

Response: "Maybe I didn't. I'm still done with it."

Notice the tone: confident-shrug energy. We're not dismissing the thought with fake positivity; we're just not taking the bait.

Keep in mind that most OCDers don't "believe" that they don't want an answer at the start. They'll tell me, "But Zach, I actually do want an answer. Saying this feels fake."

Good! It's okay that you want an answer, and it should feel fake and uncomfortable at the start because it's a new skill you're building. The point is to recognize the OCD driving you to want to have an answer, notice that urge, and then choose a different response. The longer we stick with it consistently, the less we crave an answer naturally.

Common Roadblock: "But This One's Real"

OCD *loves* this thought. Just when we've started practicing uncertainty, OCD will say, "Wait—this isn't OCD. This one feels different. You should probably solve this one. Just in case."

That's part of the cycle. We expect it to happen and we accept it.

The key is to respond with what you've learned: "This feels urgent because it's OCD. I'm not solving it. Maybe, maybe not."

Let's look at an example.

1. **Trigger/intrusive thought:** "What if I lose control and hurt someone I love?"
2. **Interpretation/meaning attached to the thought:** "This must mean I'm dangerous or broken."
3. **Recovery response option (uncertainty):** "Maybe I'm dangerous, maybe I'm not. I'll never know for sure."

Understanding Reasonable Certainty

OCD thrives on the illusion that if you just "check one more time," you'll finally feel safe. But that's not how true safety works—not with OCD, and not with life.

Let's use a common example: Health OCD and the fear of having a heart attack.

For someone without OCD, going to the doctor once a year for an annual physical and getting a routine EKG is reasonable. If something feels off, maybe they'd meet with a cardiologist just to be safe. After they're told their heart is healthy, they move on with their life. That's *reasonable certainty*.

But for someone with Health OCD, that's not where it ends. You might start going to the doctor weekly, seeking endless reassurance that you're not on the verge of a heart attack—even though multiple doctors have already told you your heart is fine. That's not reasonable anymore. That's compulsive checking. It's not based on new symptoms—it's based on fear.

And here's the trap: the very symptoms of anxiety (racing heart, tight chest, dizziness) can mimic the symptoms of a heart attack. OCD uses those sensations as "proof" that something's seriously wrong. But like we talked about, those sensations are often just your body's stress response, not a medical emergency.

There is no 100 percent certainty that any of us will never have a heart attack. But if you're healthy, have been evaluated by a medical professional, and continue to get clean bills of health, the *likelihood* is extremely low. This is where the work of recovery begins—not in finding 100 percent certainty, but in accepting reasonable certainty and living your life anyway.

OCD will always chase perfection. But peace comes when we stop chasing 100 percent and start saying, *"This is good enough. I'm choosing to trust that."*

Key Takeaway

OCD demands certainty. Recovery means choosing to live without 100 percent certainty. That choice feels scary at first, but it's the foundation of freedom. You don't have to solve the thought. You just have to stop chasing the answer.

Call to Action

Try "Maybe, Maybe Not"

For the next few days, every time a sticky thought shows up, respond with this: "Maybe it's true. Maybe it's not. I guess I'll never know for sure."

Say it with a shoulder shrug. Keep it light. You don't have to believe it right away; you just have to practice. Let your brain learn that certainty isn't required for peace.

14

INDIFFERENCE

Cool. It is what it is.

What Is Indifference?

Indifference is a behavioral stance we OCDers can take. It says, "I'm not going to react. I'm not going to try and solve this. I'm not even going to entertain this."

We don't argue with the thought.

We don't comfort ourselves.

We don't try to disprove or use logic with the thought.

We just treat it like what it is: background noise.

Here's the moneymaker we start all of our clients on: the shoulder shrug. It might seem simple, but it's incredibly powerful. A simple, physical shrug can send a clear message to our fear center: We're not taking this seriously. Our brains learn a lot from body language, and when we physically shrug off a thought, we're reinforcing the idea that it's not worth engaging with.

Even if the shrug feels fake at first, or OCD makes you feel skeptical, use it. The feeling of indifference comes later, after consistent repetition.

You're training your nervous system to stop reacting, and the shoulder shrug is one of the easiest ways to get started.

Why Indifference Works

The moment we show interest, OCD leans in. It feeds on our engagement, especially when it comes through fear, urgency, or guilt.

Indifference is the opposite of engagement. It's a way of saying, "I'm not interested today."

When indifference is practiced consistently, our brain starts to follow our lead. It learns that these thoughts don't matter because we're not reacting to them how we used to.

Over time, that reaction—or lack of it—becomes our new normal. Our brain rewires to stop overreacting.

How to Practice Indifference

Let's say you get a thought like this: "What if I want to harm someone?"

Here's what indifference sounds like:

- "Maybe I do. Maybe I don't." *(shoulder shrug)*
- "Meh." *(shoulder shrug)*
- "Not falling for that one today." *(shoulder shrug)*
- "Cool." *(shoulder shrug)*
- "Guess we'll find out." *(shoulder shrug)*
- "Oh well." *(shoulder shrug)*
- "It is what it is." *(shoulder shrug)*

Yes, some of this sounds sarcastic. That's intentional. We're leaning into a tone that robs OCD of its power.

Don't underestimate the shoulder shrug. It's a small gesture with a big impact. Our fear center takes cues from our body language, and when we shrug, we're teaching our nervous system that this isn't a big deal. Even if you feel skeptical at first, use it anyway. Once again, the body often leads the brain.

But What If It Feels Too Serious?

OCD will try to convince you that *this* thought is too dark, too serious, too real to treat with indifference.

It will say, "If you don't take this seriously, something terrible will happen, and you'll be responsible." or "If you don't take this one seriously, it's proof that you're a bad person." That's OCD talking, and it's a trap.

If we wait until the thought feels nonthreatening before we practice indifference, we'll always stay stuck. We start to reclaim our lives from OCD by first taking the action even though the feeling of fear is still there.

The shift happens *because* we choose to act indifferent in the face of discomfort. When we act indifferent enough times, the discomfort fades and we actually start to feel indifferent naturally. This gives us our freedom back.

Real Examples Across Subtypes

Harm OCD

Trigger: "What if I snap and stab someone?"
Response: "Sure, maybe." *(shoulder shrug)*

SO-OCD

Trigger: "What if I'm attracted to that person?"
Response: "Could be. Could not be. Oh well." *(shoulder shrug)*

Relationship OCD

Trigger: "What if I'm settling?"
Response: "Meh. Let's see how that plays out." *(shoulder shrug)*

Contamination OCD

Trigger: "What if I just touched something dangerous?"
Response: "Maybe I did. Guess we'll find out." *(shoulder shrug)*

Just Right OCD

Trigger: "That wasn't said perfectly."
Response: "Oh well. It is what it is." *(shoulder shrug)*

Health OCD

Trigger: "What if this pounding heart means I'm having a heart attack?"
Response: "Maybe it does. It is what it is." *(shoulder shrug)*

Let's look at an example.

1. **Trigger/intrusive thought:** "What if I lose control and hurt someone I love?"
2. **Interpretation/meaning attached to the thought:** "This must mean I'm dangerous or broken."
3. **Recovery response option (indifference):** "Maybe I am. Oh, well, it is what it is. I guess we'll see how this plays out." *(shoulder shrug)*

Key Takeaway

Indifference is powerful. It's not cold or careless. It's the choice to stop fueling fear with our attention.

We don't have to argue. We don't have to prove anything. We can just say, "Meh. It is what it is," and move on.

Now You Give It a Try

Shrug It Off

For one full day, every time an intrusive thought shows up, pause and give a calm, physical shoulder shrug. No big inner dialogue. Just a "meh" with a shoulder shrug. Notice what happens when your body starts leading the recovery response.

15

AGREEMENT

*Yep, maybe that terrible
thing is true. Oh well.*

Agreement is the tool that throws OCD off its game more than almost anything else. It's a way of saying, "Yup. You're so right. I'm a terrible person. Oh well."

Now, if that made your stomach drop a little, you're not alone. This is the most counterintuitive of all the core responses. Our brain might scream, "Wait! I can't agree with that thought! That's dangerous!"

You're not actually agreeing with the *content*. You're just taking what OCD is saying to you and giving it right back. Agreement is a way of saying, "I'm not going to try to solve this. I'm not going to argue with you anymore. If you want an answer, here's your answer."

Why Agreement Works

OCD is a master negotiator. It wants you to plead, defend, explain, argue logic, disprove, or escape. When you respond with agreement, the conversation ends. There's nothing for OCD to push against. There's no argument to escalate because you didn't give OCD anything to use.

The cycle breaks because you stop participating.

Agreement is letting go of arguing with your thoughts. It's you saying, "I don't actually need an answer on this anymore and I don't care to have one."

What Agreement Is Not

- It's not saying you want the thought to be true.
- It's not giving up or giving in.
- It's not agreeing that you actually think the thought is true.

It's a way of saying, "If that fear is true, I'll deal with it when it happens. But I'm done analyzing it."

This works because it removes urgency. It stops the compulsion. It teaches your brain to think, "We can live with this doubt. We're not afraid of it anymore."

How to Practice Agreement

Let's say you get a thought like this: "What if I'm secretly a bad person?"

Instead of pushing back, you lean in and respond with one of these statements:

- "Yep. Maybe I am."
- "Sure. Sounds about right."

- "Cool, I guess I'm just awful then."
- "Yup, I'm a total monster."
- "Maybe the worst person ever. Let's see how that goes." (You can add a shoulder shrug like you do when responding with indifference.)

The goal here isn't sarcasm for sarcasm's sake; it's disarmament. You're refusing to fuel the cycle by removing resistance.

When It Feels Wrong

OCD will fight you on this one. It'll say things like:

- "This is dangerous."
- "If you agree, it means it'll come true."
- "You're giving up your morals."

But remember, agreement is not the same as belief. You're not agreeing with the meaning. You're agreeing to stop reacting. That's where the power lies.

Real Examples Across Subtypes

Harm OCD

Trigger: "What if I snap and hurt someone?"
Response: "Sure. I'll go full psycho. Sounds like a plan."

POCD

Trigger: "What if I'm attracted to children?"
Response: "Yup. Maybe I am. Guess we'll find out."

Relationship OCD

Trigger: "What if I don't actually love my partner?"
Response: "You're so right. I don't."

Scrupulosity OCD

Trigger: "What if I sinned and didn't realize it?"
Response: "Sure. I'm probably already doomed."

Just Right OCD:

Trigger: "That didn't come out perfectly."
Response: "You're right, it didn't. Oh, well."

Health OCD

Trigger: "What if this pounding heart means I'm having a heart attack?"
Response: "Yup. This is totally a heart attack. Oh, well."

Each response is fast, clean, and deliberate. No analysis, no explanation, and no arguing. Remember, you can add a shoulder shrug as well.

The Bully on the Playground

Imagine you're back in middle school and a bully walks up to you on the playground. He starts trying to get under your skin: "Nice shirt, loser. Those shoes? Embarrassing. You probably don't even have friends."

Now imagine instead of arguing, crying, or defending yourself, you just say, "Yep. Totally agree. Worst shirt ever. Great observation. I might be the lamest person here."

The bully stares at you, confused. There's no reaction. No emotional energy to feed off. Eventually he just walks away.

That's exactly what happens when we start agreeing with OCD.

It thrives on resistance. It gets louder when we argue. When we lean in and say, "Yup, I'm absolutely the worst," it doesn't know what to do with that. There's nothing to fight.

That's when the noise starts to fade.

Let's look at an example.

1. **Trigger/intrusive thought:** "What if I lose control and hurt someone I love?"

2. **Interpretation/meaning attached to the thought:** "This must mean I'm dangerous or a horrible person."

3. **Recovery response option (agreement):** "Yep, I'm totally going to hurt someone someday. Oh, well." *(shoulder shrug)*

Choosing the Core Responses That Feel True to You

One of the most important lessons I've learned—both in my own recovery and from working with clients—is that our four core responses (acceptance, uncertainty, indifference, agreement) only work when they feel true to us. If you're just repeating a phrase because someone told you to, but it feels hollow or dishonest, it's not going to land.

For example, we had a client who struggled with harm OCD thoughts about his child. He tried saying this: "Maybe I would hurt my kid, maybe I wouldn't." But it just didn't sit right with him. Instead, he found it more genuine to say: "I don't know why this thought happens, and I'm okay with not having an answer." That phrase felt true—he genuinely didn't know, and he was learning to be okay with that uncertainty. Because he believed that response, he was able to use it consistently every time the thoughts popped up, and this created a little bit of space between him and the OCD.

Find the response that feels authentic to you. The more it resonates, the more powerfully it will help you step out of OCD's cycle.

Bonus Response: Laughter

Sometimes the best response to OCD's nonsense is laughter. Even if it feels fake or forced at first, choosing to laugh at uncomfortable thoughts sends a clear signal to our amygdala that there's no real threat. Laughter was a *huge* part of my OCD recovery journey, and it's still a staple in my life. If you can find the humor—even just a chuckle—when OCD tries to scare you, you'll teach your brain that these thoughts don't need to be taken so seriously. Give it a try. Sometimes a little laughter really is the best medicine.

Key Takeaway

Agreement is the final nail in OCD's control strategy. It says, "I'm done arguing." That's what takes the power away. You're not saying the thought is true. You're saying the thought is irrelevant and that's why you can agree with it.

Call to Action

Practice the Four Core Responses.

Take the Next Step with OCD Space

If these responses make sense on the page but feel hard to remember when you're triggered, that's normal. OCD doesn't show up on a schedule. OCD Space is a digital recovery platform where you can practice the Four Core Responses with Oscar, our clinically trained AI OCD coach, so you don't have to figure out what to say to OCD on your own.

Join OCDspace.com and start working with Oscar today

PART 4

TAKING ACTION WITH ERP

16

WHAT IS ERP?

*Do the thing you're afraid of and choose
not to do the thing that
makes it go away.*

By now, you understand the OCD cycle and how OCD works. You've learned how to shift your mindset and start responding differently with the four core responses.

Here's the next step: exposure and response prevention (ERP). It's the most effective, research-backed treatment for OCD. It's recommended by every major psychological and medical association. If you've made it this far in the book, you're already building the foundation to do it well.

Let's break it down simply. Here's what ERP stands for:

- **Exposure:** intentionally facing the thoughts, triggers, or situations that spike our anxiety
- **Response prevention:** resisting the compulsions we normally do to feel better

It's basically saying this: "I'm going to lean into this fear on purpose, and I'm not going to do any compulsions to make it go away."

It's uncomfortable and feels counterintuitive because for so long our brains have been telling us to solve the "problem." But it's the single most effective way to retrain the brain and heal from OCD.

Why ERP Works

Remember the OCD cycle? OCD throws us a thought, we panic, we compulse, and the fear gets reinforced.

ERP breaks that pattern.

When we face a trigger and don't do a compulsion, the brain gets new evidence: "We didn't do anything, and we survived. Maybe this isn't dangerous after all."

Over time, our nervous system learns that while there might not be a 100 percent guarantee, we're more than likely not in danger even if the thought is there.

ERP is not about "white-knuckling" our way through fear. It's about learning to coexist with the fear, letting it pass on its own without us needing to fix or control anything.

What Is White-Knuckling?

White-knuckling is what happens when we try to "tough it out" through an exposure by clenching our way through the discomfort. Instead of leaning into the fear with acceptance or curiosity, we grip tightly and think, "Okay, just get through this. Don't move. Don't think. Just survive it." This often looks like holding your breath, tensing your muscles, or obsessively waiting for the anxiety to go away.

For example, let's say you're doing an exposure where you touch a doorknob you fear is contaminated. If you touch it but then stand frozen, fists clenched, mentally chanting, "Don't wash your hands. Don't wash your hands"—that's white-knuckling.

While it might help you resist the compulsion in the short term, it doesn't teach your brain a new message. It reinforces the idea that the trigger *is* dangerous—you're just being "strong" enough to endure it.

Instead, we want to bring acceptance into the exposure. Relax our body. Even say to ourselves, "Yep, I feel the fear. I'm allowing it to be here."

Mindset Reminder

Discomfort Is the Path

ERP will feel uncomfortable at times—and that's okay. Discomfort is not danger. Trust the process. The goal isn't to feel better during ERP. The goal is to teach your brain that you can handle uncomfortable thoughts and feelings like fear without doing compulsions.

The Goal Isn't Less Anxiety

This is a big mindset shift. The goal of ERP is not to feel calm. The goal is to bring on the feeling of fear intentionally to train ourselves not to react with a compulsion.

Sometimes you'll do an exposure and feel less anxious afterward. Great. Other times, you'll do the same exposure and feel just as anxious or even more so. That's also okay.

Why?

Because you're teaching your brain something new by not compulsing. And that's the win. You're showing your brain that it can handle discomfort and that you don't need OCD to keep you safe anymore.

Over time and through repetition, your brain will learn not to fear that topic anymore and you won't have such a strong emotional reaction.

What ERP Looks Like in Practice

Let's say your OCD fear is "What if I hit someone with my car and didn't realize it?"

ERP might look like this:

- You drive the same route again and *don't* retrace it.
- You say out loud, "Maybe I did hit someone. It is what it is."
- You resist the urge to check news stories or police reports.
- You sit with the anxiety instead of doing mental review.

It's not about proving the thought wrong. It's about training your brain to understand you can live with the uncertainty of the thought and move forward anyway.

What ERP Is *Not*

Let's be clear:

- ERP is not flooding yourself with your worst fears all at once.
- It's not a "quick fix."
- It's not about getting rid of the thoughts or feelings.
- It's definitely not about seeking reassurance from your therapist, coach, or loved ones.

ERP is about building resilience through repeated, deliberate discomfort. It's about learning to do the opposite of what OCD wants.

ERP Isn't One-and-Done

One important thing to understand about ERP is that exposures need to be **prolonged and repetitive**. In other words, we don't just "touch the fear" for a few seconds and then run. We stay with the trigger long enough for our brain to learn, *"This is uncomfortable, but it's not dangerous."*

And we don't do exposures just once. We do them over and over again. That repetition is what rewires the brain over time. The goal isn't to prove to yourself that nothing bad will happen—it's to train your nervous system to stop treating the thought or sensation like an emergency.

A Word of Warning: OCD Will Fight Back

As you start doing ERP, expect OCD to push back. It won't go quietly.

Using the car example, let's say you drove through a crowded area and had the intrusive thought "What if I hit someone?"

OCD will try to bargain with you: "Just go back and check one time. Just this once. Then you'll be certain, and you can move on with your day. Otherwise, you'll ruminate all day."

This is the trap.

That promise of certainty is how OCD keeps us stuck. No matter how many times you check, it will never be enough. The more you give in, the more OCD demands. The next time you drive, OCD will try the same thing again. If you fall for the "just one more time" lie, you could end up doing this checking compulsion for the rest of your life.

Instead, you pause, feel the discomfort, and respond with something like this: "Maybe I did hit someone, maybe I didn't. I'm not checking. It is what it is."

That choice, that response, is how we start breaking the cycle for good.

> ## Key Takeaway
>
> ERP is how we teach our brain a new way to respond to fear. It's not about getting rid of thoughts or feelings. It's about showing up, leaning into the discomfort, and choosing not to compulse. Remember: When we pull the "C" out of OCD, the disorder fades.
>
> That's how freedom starts.

HOW ERP WORKS IN THE BRAIN

*You're not just resisting a compulsion;
you're rewiring your nervous system.*

ERP might look simple on the surface: Touch the doorknob. Don't wash your hands. Have the thought. Don't do the mental compulsion.

Under the surface, something much deeper and more powerful is happening. You're literally retraining the way your brain processes fear.

Let's walk through what that actually means.

The Fear Circuit: What's Going Wrong

With us OCDers, I always joke that our brain's threat detection system works a little too well. It's always looking for threats and it misfires a lot.

Here's how this plays out:

1. We get an intrusive thought (the trigger).
2. Our brain sounds the alarm: "Danger! This is serious!"
3. We feel panic, and we do something to try to make the feeling go away (the compulsion).

This fear circuit involves multiple brain areas, but these are the big players:

- The amygdala (responsible for fear and emotion)
- The anterior cingulate cortex (error detection—a.k.a. "something's wrong")
- The orbitofrontal cortex and caudate nucleus (decision-making and habit loops)[6]

The result is a brain that's constantly scanning for "danger," even when there's none, and then demanding we take action to neutralize or solve it.

Why ERP Changes the Game

When we do ERP, we disrupt that loop. We face the trigger, and we don't do the compulsion. We feel the anxiety, but we don't escape it.

And guess what? We teach our brains that we can handle the uncomfortable emotion and the world doesn't come crashing down.

Our brain gets new input: "Hmm . . . we didn't act on the fear, and we're still okay. Maybe this isn't an emergency after all."

This is called *inhibitory learning*. It's how the brain updates its fear files. The more often we do ERP, the stronger those new pathways become.[7] We're rewiring our brain to stop reacting to false alarms.

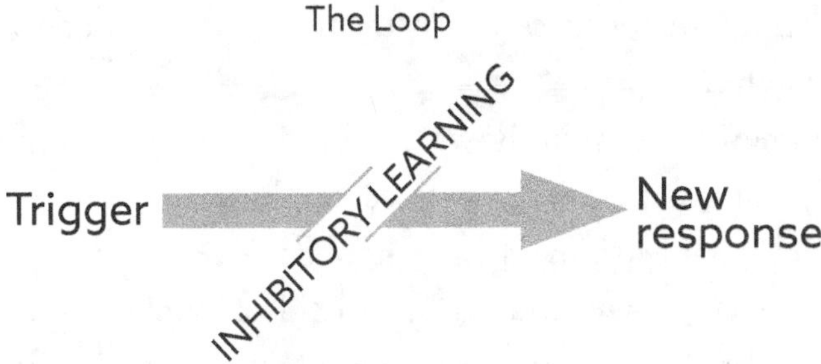

Inhibitory learning doesn't remove triggers—it changes how the brain responds when they show up.

But It Doesn't Happen All at Once

Our brain doesn't unlearn years of fear conditioning overnight. In fact, early on, it might feel like ERP isn't working: You might do an exposure and still feel anxious afterward. You might have the same intrusive thought pop up again and again. That's normal and to be expected.

You're not doing ERP to "feel better." You're doing it to teach your brain that it can survive discomfort without solving it.

That lesson takes repetition. Every time we resist a compulsion, we're laying down new neural wiring. Eventually this can lead to a decrease in intrusive thoughts and anxiety.

Habituation vs. Inhibitory Learning: What's the Difference?

For years, therapists believed that *habituation* was the main reason ERP worked. Habituation is the idea that if we expose ourselves to a feared trigger repeatedly for long enough, the anxiety will naturally fade. And for many people—including myself—it does. For example, I genuinely no longer fear SO-OCD because

I did enough exposures that I taught my brain not to fear that topic anymore.

But newer research shows there's something even more powerful happening beneath the surface: inhibitory.

Inhibitory learning is what happens when our brain builds a new association with a trigger. Instead of thinking that a trigger equals danger, the brain learns that a trigger equals discomfort—and that you can handle the discomfort.

That's a big shift.

So what does this difference actually look like?

Habituation	Inhibitory Learning
Anxiety fades with repetition	Anxiety may stay, but we respond differently
Relief is the goal	Learning is the goal
"I feel better now"	"I don't need to feel better to keep going"
Reinforces safety through exposure	Rewrites fear-based beliefs through action

Both processes can happen during ERP. Sometimes anxiety fades (habituation). Other times, it doesn't but you still grow stronger (inhibitory learning). Either way, you're winning.

The goal of ERP isn't to eliminate anxiety; it's to change our relationship with it. If you're not feeling instant relief during exposures, that's okay. That doesn't mean ERP isn't working. It means your brain is doing deeper rewiring, and it's learning that fear doesn't need a solution.

Remember: We achieve this by doing the exposure and then practicing ritual prevention. If we do an exposure but still end up compulsing afterward, we teach the brain that the ritual was necessary to stay safe—which reinforces the cycle instead of rewiring it.

Key Takeaway

ERP isn't just about behavior. It's about brain change. Every time we choose to feel the fear without feeding it, we're rewiring our threat response. We're teaching our brain to stop treating thoughts like emergencies and start treating them like background noise.

18

PREPARING FOR ERP

Courage is what happens when we do the exposure while feeling scared.

ERP is simple in theory, but doing it well takes preparation. This chapter is all about setting ourselves up for success before we dive into exposures. The more we understand what we're stepping into, the less likely we are to fall into old patterns. So let's talk about the mindset, structure, and support that will help us get the most out of ERP.

Step 1: Know Your Targets

Before we begin ERP, we need to identify what we're actually avoiding.

Start by asking these questions:

- "What thoughts make me feel the most anxious or uncertain?"

- "What situations do I avoid?"
- "What compulsions do I use to try to feel better?"

Write them down. Track them for a few days. We can't change what we haven't identified.

Step 2: Create an Exposure Hierarchy

An exposure hierarchy is a road map for ERP. It's a ranked list of feared thoughts or situations, from least scary to most scary.

Here's an example:

1. Touch a doorknob without washing hands for one minute
2. Touch a doorknob and wait ten minutes before washing
3. Touch a doorknob and don't wash at all

We're not jumping to level 10 on day one. We're gradually working up the ladder, giving our brain time to learn that it's safe to sit with uncertainty.

Harm OCD Exposure Hierarchy Example

On a scale of 1 to 10 (1 = easiest exposure, 10 = most difficult) let's develop a hierarchy for the following fear: "What if I snap and hurt someone I love?"

Here's what this might look like:

1. Read the following sentence out loud five times a day: "I could snap and hurt someone I love."
2. Look at a photo of a loved one while allowing intrusive thoughts to surface.
3. Answer the following question in your journal: "What if I lost control?" Sit with the anxiety.
4. Watch a movie scene or news clip involving someone losing control (fictional or real).

5. Write a short hypothetical script where you snap and something bad happens.

6. Record and listen to that script daily without seeking reassurance.

7. Hold an object (like a kitchen knife) alone while imagining the intrusive thought.

8. Spend time with a loved one while holding the object (with consent).

9. Hold a knife up to a loved one without compulsing (with consent).

10. Write and listen to a long script where the worst-case scenario fully plays out with you snapping and harming a loved one.

This is, of course, one specific example for one OCD subtype, but the concept applies across all themes. Please consider working with a therapist or coach if you are new to the OCD recovery process and need help creating a hierarchy.

Step 3: Expect Discomfort (and Know That's the Point)

ERP isn't supposed to feel good, but that's also why so many OCDers struggle to get started. It feels scary and challenging at the beginning, but, with time, it gets easier and easier.

When we deliberately trigger discomfort and choose not to run from it, we start to rewire the fear response. It's okay if it feels hard. It's supposed to.

And just as important: ERP only works when we practice ritual prevention. That means we don't do the behaviors that normally bring relief—no checking, reassurance, analyzing, or escaping. That's the moment the brain learns, *"I'm safe without the ritual."*

Discomfort is not a sign you're doing it wrong. It's a sign you're actually on the right path.

Step 4: Set Your Coping Responses in Advance

Before you face a fear, decide how you'll respond when anxiety shows up. Use the four core responses:

- **Acceptance:** "I'm allowing this feeling of fear to be here. It's okay."
- **Uncertainty:** "Maybe it's true, maybe it's not. I'm choosing to live with not knowing."
- **Indifference:** "Oh, well. It is what it is." *(shoulder shrug)*
- **Agreement:** "Yup, I am. Oh well." *(shoulder shrug)*
- **Nonengagement:** You can also do nothing. Allow the thought to be there and sit in it without saying anything to yourself.

Having your responses ready helps you more easily sit with discomfort—without trying to get rid of it.

Pro tip

Focus on the feeling underneath and speak to it with acceptance. Giving fear permission to be there helps drop our resistance and makes doing a compulsion less appealing.

Step 5: Get Accountability

ERP can feel scary to do alone at first. If possible, find someone who can walk with you through it—a therapist, coach, friend, or even OCDspace.com.

This isn't to get reassurance—it's to stay on track, stay honest, and stay encouraged.

Step 6: Commit to Repetition

One-and-done exposures don't create lasting change. Repetition is where the rewiring happens. We want our brain to think, "This isn't a threat. I don't need to react."

That takes practice. Daily exposures, even small ones, are what build momentum.

Think of it like going to the gym: You don't get stronger by lifting a weight once. You get stronger by showing up consistently.

Key Takeaway

ERP works best when we prepare our mindset, our plan, and our support. We're not waiting to feel ready. We're choosing to show up scared and do it anyway.

19

HOW TO DO AN EXPOSURE

The fear shows up. We show up too.
That's the work.

By now, you've built your foundation. You understand OCD. You've practiced the four core responses and talking to the OCD differently. You've prepared your exposure hierarchy. Now it's time to do the actual exposures.

This chapter will walk you through what a successful exposure looks like step-by-step.

Remember, exposures aren't about perfection. They're about participation.

A Note on Safety and Values

No exposure should ever put us in actual danger or push us out of alignment with our core values.

For example, I've heard from men struggling with sexual orientation OCD (SO-OCD) who think they need to go to a gay bar and hook up with a guy to "prove" whether they're gay.

That's not ERP. That's acting out a compulsion and trying to gain certainty.

ERP never asks us to cross boundaries that conflict with our values. It's about building tolerance for fear—not performing behaviors that cause moral or emotional distress.

A healthy in vivo exposure for SO-OCD might be looking at a picture of a man and sitting with the discomfort of an intrusive thought: "What if I felt sexually aroused?"

That's a safe, effective way to retrain the brain without violating our values.

Step 1: Choose Your Type of Exposure

There are two main types of ERP exposures:

1. **In vivo exposures:** These are real-life exposures to triggers in your external environment. You interact with something that causes fear, discomfort, or uncertainty (like touching a doorknob, not checking the stove, or driving past a school without retracing your route).

2. **Imaginal Scripting:** This involves writing or recording feared thoughts, worst-case scenarios, or triggering "what-ifs" that can't be confronted physically. They're especially useful for mental obsessions like harm OCD, SO-OCD, POCD, scrupulosity OCD, real event OCD, and false memory OCD. OCD therapists refer to this type of ERP as *imaginal scripting*, but in this book, we'll just call it *scripting*.

We'll explain how to do both types of exposures in the examples below.

Step 2: Clarify Your Goal

The goal of the exposure is not to get rid of anxiety. The goal is to feel the fear and allow it to be there without immediately doing a compulsion to get rid of it.

Remind yourself, "I'm doing this so my brain learns I can handle this discomfort. I'm not here to feel perfect."

Step 3: Lean into the Fear

Now it's time to do the exposure. Whatever the fear is, we face it head-on:

- Say the feared thought out loud: "Maybe I'll snap and hurt someone."
- Touch the doorknob and don't wash your hands.
- Look at the feared image and don't turn away.
- Write the script and listen to it on repeat for twenty minutes.

The point is to trigger anxiety on purpose and not do what OCD tells you to do to feel better. This might feel intense. That's okay. Intensity means you're in the zone where learning happens.

Step 4: Use Your Recovery Responses

As the anxiety rises, expect your brain to scream, "Fix this! Do something!"

That's your cue to use one of the four core responses:

- **Acceptance:** "I accept that this fear is here. I'm going to sit with it."
- **Uncertainty:** "Maybe it's true, maybe it's not."
- **Indifference:** "Oh, well. It is what it is." *(shoulder shrug)*
- **Agreement:** "Yep, I'm the worst." *(shoulder shrug)*

Stay present in the moment, doing your best not to white-knuckle the exposure.

Step 5: Sit with the Feeling

If it helps you to sit with the discomfort, set a timer for fifteen to thirty minutes. Remember, your job isn't to force the anxiety to go away. Your job is to stay present, not compulse, and let your brain learn that you felt the fear . . . and survived.

If your anxiety level naturally drops, that's great! If it remains relatively high, but you didn't compulse, that's great too. It means you're giving your brain the chance to rewire itself.

In Vivo Exposures (Real-World Practice)

In vivo exposures are real-life exposures to external triggers. These are actions we take in the real world that invite discomfort, fear, or uncertainty, but we don't engage in the compulsion that usually follows.

Here are six examples across different OCD subtypes:

1. **Contamination OCD:** Touch a public doorknob and resist the urge to sanitize afterward.
2. **Harm OCD:** Hold a kitchen knife while thinking, "What if I lose control and hurt someone?"
3. **Sexual orientation OCD (SO-OCD):** Look at a photo of someone of the same gender (or opposite, as applicable) and allow any uncomfortable feelings or doubts to be there.
4. **Relationship OCD (ROCD):** Look at a picture of your partner and sit with the thought "What if I don't actually love them?"
5. **Scrupulosity OCD:** Walk past a church or religious symbol without praying, repenting, or mentally apologizing.

6. **POCD:** View an image or video with children present (like a family vlog or a group photo) and allow the intrusive thought or feeling to be there without checking, analyzing, or avoiding.

These exposures may feel deeply uncomfortable. That's why they're effective. They give us the opportunity to feel the fear and choose not to compulse, which is how we teach the brain that we're safe.

How to Do Scripting Exposure

If your fear can't be confronted physically—like a thought, memory, or worst-case scenario—*scripting* is one of the most effective ways to face it head-on. It helps bring feared thoughts into the open so we can stop avoiding them and start retraining our brain.

Scripting also helps the most with rumination.

Why It Works

OCD wants us to avoid, suppress, or fix intrusive thoughts. Scripting does the opposite—it helps us say, "This fear can exist, and I can still live my life."

By exposing ourselves to the feared outcome and allowing the discomfort, we teach our brain that the thought isn't dangerous and that we don't need to neutralize it.

How to Write a Strong Script

Here's a simple framework for writing an effective script:

1. **Write in first person:** This should sound like your own voice, your own fear.
2. **Write in present tense:** "It's happening right now."

3. **Activate the trigger:** Start with a situation or thought that causes anxiety.

4. **Identify the feared outcome:** What's the worst-case scenario OCD is dangling over you?

5. **Don't include any reassurance:** No "but I'm okay, and everything ends up being fine."

6. **End with uncertainty or tragedy:** No happy endings. Leave the fear unresolved.

Script Examples

Harm OCD

I'm standing in the kitchen with a knife in my hand. I look at my partner and feel an urge to stab them. I lose control right then and hurt them. I realize I'm dangerous now and that my whole life was a lie. I go to jail and my family disowns me.

Scrupulosity OCD

I'm walking past the church, and I don't stop to pray. A voice inside tells me I just offended God. Maybe I've crossed a spiritual line and can't come back from it. Maybe I'll spend eternity disconnected, punished, and unloved. I could be doomed, and I'll never have peace again.

Sexual Orientation OCD (SO-OCD)

I walk down the street and see a man in a tight-fitting shirt, which triggers a thought: "This guy is attractive. I wonder if I could be with him." I feel a groinal response and experience what might be sexual attraction. I walk up to him, and we end up engaging in sexual acts. Afterward, I realize I don't want to be with my wife anymore, so I break up with her—even though it hurts. A few months later, my wife moves on, and I'm left with the man, feeling alone because my life has changed.

Existential OCD

I'm lying in bed staring at the ceiling when this thought hits: "What if none of this is real?" My heart starts to pound, and I can feel thoughts flooding in. "What if this is all meaningless? Maybe there's no point to any of this: relationships, accomplishments, even love. I could spend my entire life searching for purpose and never find it. Maybe everyone else is faking it too, and I'll never shake this emptiness. Maybe I'll feel this lost forever and eventually give up."

If these scripts intimidated you, that's okay. They're meant to cause uncomfortable feelings as a way to retrain our brain.

With that being said, we want to pick exposures that feel challenging but still manageable. Over time, as you build this skill, you can choose to do increasingly difficult exposures.

So, begin with easy exposures to gain momentum, just like you'd start out with light weights when you enter the world of weight training.

How to Practice Scripting

Step 1: Write, Record, and Listen

- Take five to ten minutes to write your script.
- Read it silently or out loud.
- Record it and play it back for fifteen to thirty minutes.

Step 2: Let the Anxiety Rise

- Don't avoid it. Don't analyze it.
- Allow the thoughts, feelings, images, or urges to surface.
- Don't try to distract yourself; stay focused on the script.

Step 3: Use the Four Core Responses

- **Acceptance:** "I accept this fear and thought is here."
- **Uncertainty:** "Maybe it's true, maybe it's not."
- **Indifference:** "It is what it is. Oh well." *(shoulder shrug)*
- **Agreement:** "Sure. I'm awful. Oh well." *(shoulder shrug)*

Step 4: Stay Until the Anxiety Drops by Half

- Track your anxiety from 0 to 10.
- Sit with it until it drops by half (e.g., from 8 to 4).
- This is not a hard rule but a general rule of thumb.

Step 5: Repeat Daily

- Keep using the same script until the thought feels less sticky.
- Remember that one exposure isn't enough; repetition is key.

Step 6: Repeat the Process

- Remember that OCD can shift themes, but the process for recovery remains the same.

The more you show your brain that you can sit with uncertainty and not respond, the more it rewires. Eventually, what used to spike your anxiety will barely register.

Interoceptive Exposure (Body Sensation Exposure)

This type of exposure is for when OCD latches onto physical sensations—like adrenaline, dizziness, a racing heart, shortness of breath, feeling "off," or a sense of panic. Instead of avoiding these sensations or trying to make them go away, we intentionally bring them on in a controlled way and practice not compulsing. This teaches the brain that sensations are uncomfortable but not dangerous.

Examples of interoceptive exposure include:

- Spinning in a chair for thirty to sixty seconds (to create dizziness)
- Doing jumping jacks to raise heart rate
- Breathing through a straw for thirty seconds (to trigger breath discomfort)
- Holding your breath for a short period (if medically safe)

"What If This Exposure Makes It Come True?"

This is one of the most common fears that keeps OCDers stuck: "What if doing this exposure actually causes the thing I'm afraid will happen?"

I get it. I had that exact fear too.

OCD tells us that if we do the exposure, there's a real chance we'll lose control, cause harm, or let something terrible happen.

The truth is this fear is part of the disorder. Recovery requires us to take that leap of faith, little by little, into the world of uncertainty. We don't do it all at once—we build toward uncertainty acceptance gradually. With each exposure, we teach our brain this lesson: "I can handle this. I don't need 100 percent certainty to move forward."

This is the rite of passage all of us face, and you're not alone in it.

Core Fears: Getting to the Root

OCD is a master of disguise, but underneath all the intrusive thoughts and compulsions, there's usually a core fear driving the anxiety. These core fears are universal—every one of us with OCD has at least one that feels like the deepest threat.

Researchers like Dr. Todd Pressman have identified five core fears that people experience.[8] In his work, he notes that ultimately, all fears lead to the fear of death, which makes sense—the brain's job is to keep us alive and safe.

The Five Core Fears

1. **Loss of love:** This is fear of rejection, abandonment, or being unloved. "If people knew what I was thinking, they'd leave me."
2. **Loss of identity:** This is fear of not knowing who you are or being someone "bad." "What if I'm not who I thought I was?"
3. **Loss of meaning:** This is fear that life is pointless or empty. "What if none of this matters?"
4. **Loss of purpose:** This is fear that you'll never achieve or contribute anything. "What if I'm never good enough or don't make a difference?"
5. **Loss of life (death):** This is the ultimate fear—physical death or annihilation. "What if I die or someone I love dies?"

Two other core fears I see a lot in OCD are the fear of ending up alone and unwanted forever, and the fear of being hopelessly unhappy. These fears can feel especially real in themes like relationship OCD, existential OCD, or depression-linked

OCD—where OCD tries to convince us that life will never feel normal again.

Using Core Fears in Scripts

When you're creating a script for exposure, it can help to go deeper—right to the core fear. Here are some examples of how to do that:

- If you fear harming someone (loss of love), you might write, "I hurt someone and everyone I care about leaves me."
- If you fear making a mistake at work (loss of purpose), your script could be, "I fail, lose my job, and never find my way."

How to Find Your Core Fear: The Downward Arrow Technique

If you're not sure what your core fear is, try the downward arrow technique. Here's an example:

1. Start with your surface fear: "What if I made a mistake?"
2. Ask, "If that were true, why would that be so bad?" Answer, "People would think I'm incompetent."
3. Ask, "And if that happened, why would that be bad?" Answer, "I'd lose my job."
4. Ask, "And why would that be bad?" Answer, "I'd disappoint my family."
5. Ask, "And why would that be bad?" Answer, "I'd be alone, and my life wouldn't matter."

In this example, we can see that person's initial fear of making a mistake isn't actually what he's afraid of. Deep inside, he is afraid that mistakes will lead to people abandoning him, which is loss of love. This technique will usually illuminate your core fear.

Don't Stress If You're Unsure

If you don't know exactly which core fear is at play, that's okay! Many of us have a blend of them, and the lines aren't always clear.

The important thing is to be curious, not perfect. The point of knowing your core fear is to incorporate it into your script so you can take it a layer deeper. But knowing your core fear is not a requirement, so please don't get hung up on this if you're unsure. Scripts can still be effective without the core fear present.

Key Takeaway

Exposures aren't about eliminating fear. They're about teaching your brain that fear isn't a threat. The more we face the fear and choose not to compulse, the less power OCD has over our lives.

Want Help Crafting Your Scripts?

If doing ERP on your own feels overwhelming or confusing, you're not alone. OCD Space was built to support people through the ERP process at their own pace. When I started ERP, I remember how isolating and uncertain it felt—and I built Oscar to be the kind of support I wish I'd had then.

Oscar, our clinically trained AI OCD coach, can help you think through hypothetical scripts, plan exposures, and stay aligned with recovery principles without turning ERP into reassurance.

Scan the QR code or visit OCDspace.com to get started

20

REAL-LIFE ERP EXAMPLES

*Courage is facing fear,
not the absence of fear.*

If you're anything like I was at the start of my recovery, ERP can feel overwhelming. You hear phrases like "trigger your worst fear" or "sit in uncertainty," and your brain instantly panics: "I can't do that. It's too much."

The truth is *you already do ERP all the time*, just in the wrong direction.

Every time you avoid a trigger, you're doing ERP in reverse. You're teaching your brain that the fear is real and must be escaped.

This chapter is here to flip that and show you what it looks like when you walk *toward* the fear instead.

These are real examples and real exposures from real people reclaiming their lives.

Contamination OCD—Matthew

Fear: "If I don't wash my hands enough, someone I love will get sick and die."

Compulsion: Washing hands over twenty times a day. avoiding shared surfaces.

Exposure: Touched a public doorknob, then ate lunch without washing hands.

Response prevention: No washing. No Googling. No asking for reassurance.

What he learned: "I didn't get sick. No one else did either. The anxiety passed. I can accept that getting sick is a possibility, but more than likely it won't happen."

ROCD—Sarah

Fear: "What if I don't really love my partner and I'm just settling?"

Compulsion: Comparing feelings, checking past memories, rumination.

Exposure: Wrote a script about herself and her partner breaking up.

Response prevention: No analyzing. No testing. No outside validation.

What she learned: "I didn't need to feel perfectly in love to stay present. I started showing up without needing constant proof."

Health OCD—Taylor

Fear: "What if I have a hidden illness and don't catch it in time?"

Compulsion: Googling symptoms, frequent doctor visits, body scanning.

Exposure: Canceled all nonessential appointments and wrote a script imagining her worst-case health fear coming true.

Response prevention: No Googling. No checking. No reassurance from others.

What she learned: "Sitting with the fear helped my brain see that fear isn't danger. I can live with uncertainty."

Self-Harm OCD—Carter

Fear: "What if I secretly want to hurt myself?"

Compulsion: Avoiding knives, mental checking, reassurance-seeking.

Exposure: Wrote a script where he snapped, harmed himself, and others couldn't save him. Listened to it daily.

Response prevention: No reassurance. No reviewing. No resisting the thought.

What he learned: "The thought lost its grip the more I let it be there. I stopped proving I was safe and accepted that it's okay that I have these thoughts from time to time."

SO-OCD—Kathryn

Fear: "What if I'm gay and don't know it?"

Compulsion: Scanning for groinal responses, reviewing memories, comparing people.

Exposure: Wrote scripts of her sexual orientation suddenly changing.

Response prevention: No bodychecking. No analyzing. No comparing.

What she learned: "I didn't need certainty; I needed to stop chasing it."

POCD—Tori

Fear: "What if I'm a danger to children?"

Compulsion: Avoiding kids, mentally reviewing past moments, Googling POCD.

Exposure: Wrote a script of her worst fear playing out and listened to it daily.

Response prevention: No reassurance. No checking her body's reaction. No distraction.

What she learned: "The point wasn't to make the thought go away. It was to show my brain it didn't matter."

Existential OCD—Andrew

Fear: "What if life has no meaning and nothing matters?"

Compulsion: Rumination, excessive research, avoidance of quiet time.

Exposure: Recorded a script where life was meaningless and hopeless. Listened to it every day without trying to feel better.

Response prevention: No Googling. No solving. No mental debate.

What he learned: "I didn't need the answer, I needed to stop needing one."

Small Exposures = Big Wins

Not every exposure needs to be dramatic. Sometimes it's texting someone without rereading it twelve times. Sometimes it's walking past a triggering area and allowing your thoughts to just be there. Every exposure counts.

How Long Should You Do Exposure Work?

The length of intentional exposure work varies from person to person, but here's what I've found most helpful for myself and clients I've worked with over the years.

For most, a focused "exposure blitz" period of three to six months builds serious momentum and rewires the brain's response to fear. During this period, you do some form of intentional exposure every day.

After that, exposure work usually shifts to an as-needed basis.

To this day, I still do exposures whenever OCD tries to flare up, but it's no longer a daily routine. Instead, my regular toolbox includes daily or weekly habits like exercise, meditation, good sleep, the letting go technique, and the four core responses.

Everyone's journey is different, so listen to your needs and pace yourself.

Key Takeaway

Every ERP example has two parts:

1. Facing the fear

2. Letting go of the urge to fix it

You don't need to be perfect. You just need to be willing.

21

THE BIGGEST ERP PITFALL

If you're doing the exposure but still doing the compulsion, you're not retraining the brain.

ERP is one of the most powerful tools we have for OCD recovery. But like any tool, it only works if we use it correctly.

One of the biggest mistakes we OCDers make in ERP is that we do the exposure, but we don't actually *stop doing the compulsion*.

Maybe we resist the compulsion on the surface, but underneath, we're white-knuckling it—gritting our teeth, clenching our jaw, counting the seconds until the anxiety passes.

I get it because I've been there.

As you learned earlier, white-knuckling is still a form of resistance, and resistance keeps the fear alive.

What White-Knuckling Looks Like

White-knuckling doesn't always look dramatic. It can be subtle, like mentally chanting a mantra to feel safe, subtly distracting yourself, or obsessively checking to see if the anxiety is going down.

Here's what it might sound like:

- "Okay, I'm doing the exposure, but when is this going to go away?"
- "I just have to make it through this and then I'll feel better."
- "This better work or I'm screwed."

And underneath all of that? Here's what we're experiencing:

- A hidden need to feel relief
- A quiet demand for certainty
- A subtle compulsion still being fed

Which means OCD is still in control.

Why It Doesn't Work

When we white-knuckle our way through ERP, the brain doesn't learn that we're safe. It learns, "I'm still in danger, but now I'm not even allowed to protect myself."

Instead of rewiring fear, you just exhaust your nervous system and reinforce the belief that anxiety equals an emergency.

What to Do Instead: True Response Prevention

Real ERP isn't about forcing yourself through the fear. It's about learning to let the fear be there without trying to fix it.

Here's how to approach ERP more effectively:

- **Expect discomfort** and welcome it. ("Of course this feels hard. I expected this. I can do hard things.")
- **Stay with the feeling,** not the thought. ("This anxiety is allowed to be here.")
- **Drop the stopwatch.** Don't chase relief. ("It'll pass when it passes.")
- **Use the four core responses** to neutralize the thought instead of engaging with it.

My Own Biggest Pitfall: "I Can't Be Happy Until the Thoughts Are Gone"

At the start of my own OCD journey, I repeated one phrase to myself constantly: "I can't be happy until I never have another intrusive thought ever again."

In my mind, intrusive thoughts were "bad," and bad meant I was either a horrible person or my worst fear was going to come true. I didn't realize it at the time, but that belief system was sending a message to my brain: "These thoughts are unacceptable. You're not allowed to have them."

As a result, I couldn't fully accept them. I couldn't be uncertain about them, be indifferent to them, or agree with them. Because deep down, I believed that just having an intrusive thought meant something was wrong with me.

So I stayed stuck.

Until one day, it clicked: The problem wasn't the intrusive thoughts; it was my relationship to them.

I had convinced myself that freedom meant never thinking the thoughts again. But that belief was what kept me trapped. Every time one popped up, it felt like I had failed.

So I changed my goal. I stopped aiming to never have an intrusive thought again.

I started aiming to never *fear* an intrusive thought again. I wanted to get to a place where I could have an intrusive thought and say, "So what? Oh well." I wanted them to pass like junk content in my mental inbox—noticed, maybe, but not opened or obsessed over.

That shift changed everything. To this day, I still have intrusive thoughts. The difference is I don't really care. I don't remember most of them. I don't give them weight.

I shrug. I use one of my four core responses, and I keep moving forward.

Challenge Your Belief System

If you're telling yourself you can't be happy until the thoughts go away, I want to challenge that.

Try this instead: "What if my real freedom comes from not caring about the thoughts anymore?"

That shift is the difference between feeling stuck and feeling free. And that freedom is available to you starting today.

Rewarding Ourselves After Exposure Work

Exposure work can feel hard. It takes courage, energy, and vulnerability. That's why it's so important that we reward ourselves for showing up and doing the work even if it was uncomfortable or didn't feel "perfect."

Building in rewards helps motivate our brains, shifts recovery from "just another chore" to something more positive, and keeps us moving forward. The trick is to pick rewards that genuinely excite you—something you'll actually look forward to.

Here are a few ideas:

- Binge a favorite TV show after your exposure session.
- Go out for ice cream or your favorite treat.
- Book a massage or spa day as a bigger reward for hitting a milestone.
- Take yourself to a movie, to a new coffee shop, or on a nature walk.
- Download a new book or album you've been wanting.
- Call a friend or family member to celebrate your progress.

Recovery is serious work, but that doesn't mean we can't make it enjoyable along the way. The more you reinforce the positives, the more likely you are to stick with it for the long haul. You deserve to celebrate every single win, big or small.

Key Takeaway

ERP isn't about white-knuckling your way to relief. It's about changing your relationship to the thoughts so they no longer control your behavior.

Let go of the goal to feel "better." Replace it with the goal to build resilience—and see how everything changes.

What's Next

Letting Go of the Fear

If you're wondering, "Okay, but how do I actually allow myself to feel feelings?"—that's exactly what we're going to explore next.

I'll introduce you to the *letting go technique*, inspired by the powerful work of Dr. David R. Hawkins. It's a practice that's helped me (and so many of the clients we've worked with) finally let go of the fear underneath the thoughts. This is achieved not by fixing them but by feeling the emotion that drives them. It's the next layer of recovery. It's what makes ERP not just effective but transformational.

Let's dive in.

PART 5

LETTING GO

Up to this point, we've covered the foundation of OCD recovery: understanding the cycle, resisting compulsions, and using ERP. That's the core of evidence-based treatment—and it works.

So you might be wondering why I'm including a section on the letting go technique. The reason is simple: recovery isn't just about what we *do* on paper. It's about how we handle discomfort, emotions, and uncertainty in real time—especially when **OCD** feels loud.

This section isn't meant to replace ERP. It's meant to support it by giving you another skill to stop fighting your internal experience and return to the only thing that matters: Responding differently and continuing to live your life.

22

THE LETTING GO TECHNIQUE

"To let go of a feeling involves a decision to stop holding on to it. It means to release it, to acknowledge it, to be aware of it, and to allow it to run its course."

—DR. DAVID R. HAWKINS

Discovering *Letting Go: The Pathway of Surrender* by Dr. David Hawkins was the missing piece in my recovery. I understood ERP. I was working the mindset shifts and using tools like meditation. But I still found myself getting frustrated by one specific part of the process: the feelings.

What I didn't realize was that underneath all the thoughts, all the stories I told myself, there were emotions I was still resisting and hadn't processed. The more I resisted those emotions, the more stuck my emotions became.

Dr. Hawkins's work changed that. His technique gave me a framework for what it actually means to let go of emotional resistance, and it's something I still use to this day.

If ERP is the physical muscle of recovery, letting go is the emotional one.

Under Every Thought Is a Feeling

This is something that isn't talked about enough in OCD recovery: Every intrusive thought has an underlying emotion that OCDers are trying to avoid.

Take a second and think about it. Underneath all the thoughts you're having is an emotion. You might be having thoughts of harming someone, contaminating your hands, not being your sexual orientation, or being a bad partner. Underneath the thought is the real driver: fear, guilt, shame, grief, frustration, or pride.

Here's an example:

- You think, "What if I hurt someone?"
- Your chest tightens. Your hands sweat, and you feel panic.
- Your brain tells you, "Fix this. Figure this out. Do something."

What's really happening is that you're trying to escape the emotion underneath the thought. This is where the letting go technique becomes your greatest ally.

What Is the Letting Go Technique?

Letting go is not about *getting rid of* a thought or emotion. It's about surrendering to it. It's about allowing the feeling to move through us, without trying to change, suppress, or control it.

Here's how Dr. Hawkins explains it in *Letting Go*: "To let go of a feeling involves a decision to stop holding on to it. To stop resisting it. To stop giving it energy."[9]

The reason a feeling stays stuck is because we judge it, fear it, or try to fix it. When we drop the resistance, the emotion is free to pass. You can think of this like white-knuckling. The more we resist the emotion, the more strength we give it.

"But I'm Afraid If I Let Go, It Will Come True"

One of the most common fears people express when learning this technique is "But if I stop thinking about it, what if it actually happens? If I let go of the fear, isn't that irresponsible?"

This is OCD's favorite lie, and it keeps so many of us locked in endless problem-solving and ritualizing. We're convinced that the only thing keeping us (or others) safe is our worry. But underneath this fear is a deeper emotional truth.

When we say, "I can't let this go," here's what we're often really feeling:

- **Fear:** "I don't trust myself or the world."
- **Guilt:** "If I stop thinking about it, something bad might happen and it will be my fault."
- **Shame:** "Letting go means I'm a bad person who doesn't care."

These are the emotions OCD latches on to. Our mind, trying to escape them, starts compulsively problem-solving the emotions by trying to think its way out of the feeling.

Letting go asks something radically different: "Am I courageous enough to stop problem-solving this feeling and allow it to be here?"

It's about sitting with discomfort—not because we've fixed it but because we've finally stopped running from it.

This isn't about being reckless or careless. It's about building the emotional muscle to say, "I'm willing to feel this. I'm willing to stop fighting it. I'm willing to stop trying to figure it out."

That's not passivity. That's power.

Suppression, Repression, and the Emotional Build-Up

Dr. Hawkins teaches that most of us, whether we realize it or not, are walking around with years (sometimes decades) of unfelt, unprocessed emotion trapped in our system from various life events, including traumatic ones.

According to his model, this translates to two responses:

- **Suppression** is when we consciously push feelings away. We tell ourselves things like "I don't have time to deal with this" or "Just move on."
- **Repression** is when the mind unconsciously blocks emotions from awareness, usually because they were too overwhelming when we first experienced them.

Over time, both lead to emotional residue, which is a build-up in the body and nervous system. It's like trying to hold dozens of inflated beach balls underwater at once. Eventually, the pressure builds and something has to give.

That's where OCD comes in. OCD feeds on this emotional pressure.

When there's a backlog of unprocessed fear, guilt, sadness, or shame, intrusive thoughts latch on like magnets. The brain uses thoughts to try to "solve" the feeling, when really, what needs to happen is simple: We need to let the emotion come up, be felt, and move through us.

Letting go allows that release to happen.

When we allow emotions to come up and pass through, we feel lighter, more peaceful, and more present. OCD loses the emotional fuel it needs to survive.

That's why this technique isn't just a mindset shift; it's a full-body reset.

How to Practice Letting Go (the Hawkins Method)

Here's the process, step-by-step:

1. Locate the Feeling in the Body

Redirect your attention from the thoughts in your head to what's happening in your body. Where is the sensation? Chest? Stomach? Throat? Let it be there.

2. Allow the Feeling to Exist Without Resistance

Don't label it. Don't try to breathe it away. Just sit with it. Let it be intense if it wants to be. This is *emotional exposure*, and it's safe.

3. Drop the Mental Story

Let go of the thought loop. You don't need to solve, analyze, or explain. You're just here to feel. "I don't need to figure this out. I'm going to allow this feeling to be here."

4. Stay Present

Bring gentle attention to your breath or to the part of your body where the feeling lives. Watch the sensation rise, peak, and eventually pass.

Why Letting Go Works in OCD Recovery

OCD is a fight response. We fight the thoughts. We fight the feelings. We fight to stay in control.

Letting go ends the fight.

When we stop resisting the emotion that OCD is trying to bait us into avoiding, we reclaim our power. We're no longer afraid of the feeling, so the thought loses its grip.

Here's what it sounds like: "This feeling can be here. I'm okay with it."

This is how we move from compulsive urgency to courage and confidence.

With Gratitude

This technique is entirely based on the work of Dr. David R. Hawkins, whose book *Letting Go: The Pathway of Surrender* has changed countless lives, including mine.

If you resonate with this chapter, I strongly encourage you to read or listen to the full book. It's one of the most important texts I've ever come across.

Key Takeaway

Letting go isn't about getting rid of emotions. It's about feeling them fully, without resistance, so they can move through us and lose their grip.

When we surrender the fight, we stop feeding OCD. When we focus on the feeling underneath the thoughts we're experiencing, we allow the feeling to move through us. The thoughts can then become less frequent or disappear altogether. Read the next chapter to learn how to apply the letting go technique in your life.

23

LETTING GO IN REAL LIFE

---

*"Surrender is the simple but profound
wisdom of yielding to rather than
opposing the flow of life."*

—DR. DAVID R. HAWKINS

It's one thing to understand letting go as a concept. It's another thing entirely to apply it in real life, when your chest is tight, your mind is spinning, and OCD is screaming for attention.

That's what this chapter is about: practicing the letting go technique in your day-to-day life.

Letting go is a skill we use daily *as life is happening.* When the intrusive thoughts come and the discomfort shows up, we deploy our skills.

This is where Dr. Hawkins's work becomes even more powerful. It gives us a *map* of human emotions. A road map that shows us exactly what's going on beneath the surface.

The Emotional Frequency Chart (Map of Consciousness)

Dr. Hawkins developed what he called the Map of Consciousness—a chart that organizes emotions by their energetic frequency. Each emotional state has a vibration, and that vibration influences how we feel, think, and behave.

Here's a simplified version of the chart:

Emotion	Frequency	State
Shame	20	Humiliation
Guilt	30	Blame
Apathy	50	Despair
Grief	75	Regret
Fear	100	Anxiety
Desire	125	Craving
Anger	150	Frustration, resentment
Pride	175	Judgment, ego
Courage	**200**	**Willingness to face**
Neutrality	250	Flexibility, trust
Willingness	310	Openness
Acceptance	350	Understanding
Love	500	Compassion, unity
Peace	600	Inner stillness
Enlightenment	700+	Transcendence

Everything below 200 is considered a *contracted state*—survival mode. Everything at 200 or above is an *expansive state*, where healing and flow begin to emerge.

Most of us with OCD live in the lower frequencies, especially fear, guilt, and shame. Letting go doesn't mean forcing ourselves into higher frequencies. It means releasing what we're holding on to so we can *naturally* rise into higher frequencies.

Can you identify which emotion(s) you've been operating from lately?

Real-World Emotion Breakdowns (and How to Let Them Go)

Let's walk through how each of these emotions shows up for us in OCD—and what surrendering them actually looks like.

Shame (Frequency: 20)

- **What it feels like:** worthlessness, "I'm broken," self-isolation
- **Behavior it drives:** hiding, withdrawing, denying support
- **Letting go of shame:**
  - Offer yourself compassion.
  - Say, "This feeling doesn't define me. I'm choosing to feel it and release it."

Guilt (Frequency: 30)

- **What it feels like:** heavy, shameful, "I must be a bad person"
- **Behavior it drives:** mental reviewing, apologizing, confessing
- **Letting go of guilt:**
  - Acknowledge it without judgment.
  - Say, "I release the need to punish myself. I allow this feeling to pass."

Grief (Frequency: 75)

- **What it feels like:** heaviness, mourning the "old me," hopelessness
- **Behavior it drives:** avoidance, despair, loss of motivation
- **Letting go of grief:**
  - Let the sadness be there, without rushing to escape it.
  - Say, "This grief is here because I care. I give myself permission to feel it."

Fear (Frequency: 100)

- **What it feels like:** racing heart, intrusive thoughts, a sense of urgency, "what-ifs"
- **Behavior it drives:** compulsions, checking, avoiding, reassurance-seeking
- **Letting go of fear:**
  - Notice the fear in your body.
  - Let go of the urge to "solve" the thought.
  - Say "This fear is here, and that's okay. I allow myself to feel it."

Anger (Frequency: 150)

- **What it feels like:** irritation at OCD, frustration with the process, "Why me?"
- **Behavior it drives:** snapping at others, giving up, self-sabotage
- **Letting go of anger:**
  - Sit with the anger without acting on it.
  - Say, "I'm angry, and I'm choosing to feel it without reacting."

Pride (Frequency: 175)

- **What it feels like:** ego defense, denial, "I shouldn't be struggling"
- **Behavior it drives:** hiding symptoms, resisting support, perfectionism
- **Letting go of pride:**
    - Acknowledge that pride may be covering deeper pain.
    - Say, "I don't have to have it all together. I'm allowed to ask for help."

Why Guilt and Shame Keep Us Stuck

Dr. Hawkins identified shame and guilt as the lowest-vibrating emotional states on the human consciousness scale. Shame vibrates at 20. Guilt at 30. Both keep us trapped in suffering, isolation, and self-rejection.

For many of us with OCD, these feelings show up constantly. OCD tells us we're dangerous. Broken. Bad.

And in an attempt to prove that we're *not* those things, we hold on to guilt and shame—consciously or unconsciously—as a way to "atone." We think, "If I feel bad enough, maybe it proves I'm a good person."

That's a trap.

Holding on to guilt or shame doesn't make us better. It just keeps us stuck in the loop. The most healing thing we can do is this: Feel the feeling. Acknowledge it. And *let it go.*

For example, we can let go of needing to prove we're a good person. The need to "prove" something is keeping the guilt and OCD loop alive. If we're willing to let go of this, we find the feeling of guilt eventually passes on its own, as the brain no longer needs it to justify that we're a good person.

Interestingly, when previous clients of mine let go of guilt associated with being a "bad person," they start to naturally feel like good people. They report feeling lighter, more joyous, and they experience better social interactions with others.

Letting Go = Courage

On Hawkins's scale, 200—courage—is the gateway to healing.

It's not about eliminating fear. It's about saying, "I'm willing to feel this. I'm no longer running."

When we move into courage, we signal to our brains that we are willing to feel fear and not run from it anymore. We start to feel fear courageously. That's where OCD starts to lose its grip.

Practicing Letting Go in the Moment

Letting go is a real-time skill. Here's a common scenario:

1. **Trigger:** You see a knife and think, "What if I snap and hurt someone?"
2. **Emotion:** Your heart pounds. You feel fear, guilt, maybe even shame.
3. **Letting go response:**
   - Become aware of the feeling underneath the thought.
   - Move attention to the body.
   - Let the emotion rise without compulsing.
4. **Release:** Eventually, the wave passes. You didn't analyze or fix it. You surrendered. That's real healing.

The Power of Staying with a Feeling

One of the biggest mindset shifts in letting go is this: You're not trying to get rid of the feeling. You're trying to stay with it long enough for it to release on its own.

When an emotion rises, the mind immediately wants to fix, modify, soothe, or analyze it. We want to do *something* to make it go away.

Healing happens when we do the opposite.

Letting go means making a conscious commitment to stay with the feeling without reacting, suppressing, or distracting, until it naturally passes through. That might take thirty seconds. It might take ten minutes. The timeline isn't the point. The point is that you're trusting your body to do what it knows how to do—process emotion.

Say to yourself, "I'm willing to feel this. I'm staying with it. I don't need to change it. I just need to let it process on its own time."

This is where the real magic happens. This is how emotions stop recycling and start resolving.

How to Practice the Letting Go Technique (Formally)

You don't need hours of free time or a quiet retreat to release stuck emotions. You just need a few minutes of intentional presence.

Here's how to do a formal letting go practice using Dr. David Hawkins's questions.

Set the Scene

- Find a quiet place.
- Lie down or sit comfortably.
- Close your eyes.
- Set a timer for ten to fifteen minutes.

Bring a Topic to Mind

Think of a situation, thought, or memory that's been stirring up uncomfortable emotions—fear, guilt, sadness, shame, etc. Allow the images, thoughts, urges, and sensations around it to bubble up without trying to change or fix them.

Ask These Seven Questions Gently in Order

Ask each one slowly, without pressure or the expectation that you must feel a certain way. Just be curious and open.

1. **What am I feeling right now?** (Identify the emotion—fear, sadness, guilt, etc.)
2. **Could I allow myself to feel this feeling?** (Not force it away—just allow it.)
3. **Could I welcome it in?** (Can you allow even just a little more openness?)
4. **Could I drop my resistance to feeling it?** (Am I clenching against it? Can I soften?)
5. **Could I let it go?** (Could I allow it to pass through naturally?)
6. **Would I be willing to let it go?** (Is there a willingness to surrender, even a tiny bit?)
7. **When?** (Right now is always an option.)

It's okay if the answer to a question is no. Simply answer yes or no—without judging or analyzing—and move on to the next one. No need to linger or "make" something happen. Just keep flowing through the process. Simply going through the process begins the natural unwinding of suppressed or repressed emotions.

Repeat Three to Four Rounds

Choose the same emotion or topic and gently cycle through the questions again. With each round, you may feel the emotion begin to soften or shift.

How Do I Know I'm Doing the Letting Go Technique Correctly?

This is one of the most common questions I get, and it makes sense. If you're like most of us with OCD, you're used to constantly checking, evaluating, and needing to "get it right."

Let me offer you some relief: There's no perfect way to do the letting go technique.

Letting go isn't about controlling the feeling. It's not about trying to "make it go away." It's simply about allowing it to be there—without resistance.

Here's what letting go *does* look like:

- You pause instead of reacting or compulsing.
- You identify the emotion under the thought (fear, guilt, shame, etc.).
- You bring your awareness to the sensation in your body.
- You breathe into it and say, "I'm willing to feel this. I don't need to change it."
- You stay with it—without trying to suppress, analyze, or fix it.

If you're doing those things, you're doing it right. Even if it feels uncomfortable. Even if the emotion doesn't go away immediately. Releasing is not about forcing an outcome; it's about making peace with whatever shows up.

How Will I Know When a Release Happens?

A release can look and feel different for everyone. Some people describe it as follows:

- A wave of calm
- A physical softening (shoulders drop, breath deepens)

- A sensation of energy moving or dissolving
- A subtle sense of emotional lightness
- A sudden insight or moment of clarity

But here's the key: You don't have to chase the release. In fact, trying to force a release becomes a form of control, and control is OCD's game.

Think of letting go like unclenching your fist. Sometimes, you'll feel the shift instantly. Other times, it happens quietly, gradually, like a knot unraveling over time.

Trust the process. Each time you willingly feel instead of fight, you're releasing, even if the evidence doesn't show up right away.

What Surrender Really Means

In the context of letting go, surrender doesn't mean giving up. It doesn't mean giving in to OCD. It doesn't mean agreeing with your thoughts or resigning yourself to suffering.

Surrender simply means this: "I'm going to stop fighting this moment."

You're letting go of the mental battle and the need to control what you're thinking or feeling. You're allowing the experience to unfold without compulsions, without judgment, and without force.

It's the difference between clenching your fists and opening your hands.

Surrender is not weakness. It's a powerful, conscious decision to stop feeding the loop.

When we stop resisting, we create the space for the thoughts and feelings to pass.

Mourning the Old You—and Why That's Okay

A common part of OCD recovery is the grief that comes with it. You might find yourself mourning who you were *before* the OCD spiked. Before the thoughts. Before the panic. Before the seemingly endless rituals and spirals.

That grief is real, and it's valid.

You're not just letting go of compulsions. You're letting go of a version of yourself that felt more carefree.

Here's what's actually happening: The old version of you wasn't more whole, it was just less aware of what was happening inside your nervous system. Now is an opportunity to feel your feelings fully and deploy the letting go technique.

Allow yourself to feel the sadness. Allow yourself to miss the "old" version of you. Then, when you're ready, allow the sadness to be fully felt and move through you.

The mourning of your old self might not pass in a second or a minute, but if you stay in the mindset of allowing the feeling to be there without judgment, it will eventually pass. I know this because I mourned my "old self" too, and the letting go technique allowed me to fully feel and process the emotion before choosing to let it go on my own time, once I was ready.

You're growing into a new version of yourself. One that's stronger, more grounded, and more equipped than ever before. Even if you can't see it yet, it's happening.

The mourning is part of the healing. You're not going backward; you're making space for something new.

Key Takeaway

You don't need to feel good to let go. You just need to *stop resisting* what you're already feeling.

Letting go creates the space for emotions like fear to pass on their own. When we stop fueling thoughts with underlying emotions, OCD starts to fade.

Take the Next Step with OCD Space

If letting go feels confusing at first, that's completely normal. This isn't a skill you master by thinking harder—it's something you learn through practice, over time.

That's why I built OCD Space and Oscar. When you're unsure how to let go in a specific moment, Oscar-our clinically trained AI OCD coach, can help you slow things down, see where you might be getting stuck, and guide you back to a recovery-aligned response.

Join OCDspace.com and start working with Oscar today

24

REAL-LIFE LETTING GO EXAMPLES

"We surrender a feeling by allowing it to be there without condemning, judging, or resisting it. We simply look at it, observe it, and allow it to be felt without trying to modify it. With the willingness to relinquish a feeling, it will run out in due time."

—DR. DAVID R. HAWKINS

By now, you've learned what letting go is, how it works, and how it can be practiced in real time. If you're anything like me, hearing a concept isn't enough. You want to see it in action. This chapter is here to show you exactly how letting go looks and feels in real-world OCD situations.

The Setup: It's Not About the Thought

Remember, letting go isn't about arguing with the thought. It's about feeling the emotion underneath it and giving it space to pass on its own.

For every story below, the thought might be different, but the pattern is the same:

- The trigger arises.
- A wave of emotion floods in.
- The choice is made to feel it, not fix it.

Harm OCD Example: "What if I snap and hurt someone I love?"

1. **Trigger:** Kim sees a kitchen knife and thinks, "What if I lose control and stab my partner?"
2. **Emotional reaction:** A surge of fear, followed by guilt and shame.
3. **Old response:** Avoid the kitchen, hide the knives, mentally review every past moment for reassurance.
4. **Letting go response**
   a. She pauses.
   b. She notices the fear in her chest and stomach.
   c. She names it: "I'm feeling fear. And I'm willing to let it be here."
   d. She doesn't suppress it. She doesn't try to solve the thought.
   e. She sets a timer for ten minutes and goes through the letting go technique.
5. **Release:** The emotion peaks and then passes. Not because she "figured it out" but because she let herself feel the emotion of fear without resisting.

Relationship OCD Example: "What if I don't love my partner enough?"

1. **Trigger:** Christian is cuddling his wife and suddenly thinks, "What if this means I don't love her?"
2. **Emotional reaction:** Guilt, grief, and a desperate craving for certainty.
3. **Old response:** Mental reviewing, comparing feelings to past relationships, asking for reassurance.
4. **Letting go response:**
   a. He closes his eyes.
   b. He notices the tightness in his chest and the urge to think.
   c. He chooses instead to feel the emotion directly.
   d. He says, "I welcome this guilt. I let go of the need to solve this right now."
5. **Release:** He sits with it—no analysis, no reaction. Just feeling. With each repetition of this practice, his need to solve the thought loosens.

Existential OCD Example: "What if life is meaningless?"

1. **Trigger:** Owen is walking alone and suddenly thinks, "What if nothing matters?"
2. **Emotional reaction:** A deep wave of grief, fear, and sadness.
3. **Old response:** Spiraling into philosophical analysis, watching YouTube videos on the meaning of life, trying to escape the void.
4. **Letting go Response:**
   a. He places his hand on his chest.
   b. He feels the sadness, not as a concept but as energy moving through his body.
   c. He breathes into it.

    d. He says, "I'm willing to feel this emptiness. I'm letting go of having to solve it."

5. **Release:** The feeling rises, peaks, and fades. He doesn't feel "fixed," but he feels more grounded, more present, and less controlled by the thought.

SO-OCD Example: "What if I'm actually gay and don't know it?"

1. **Trigger:** Ethan sees a guy at the gym and thinks, "What if I'm attracted to him? What if I'm gay and living a lie?"

2. **Emotional reaction:** A rush of fear, followed by shame and an overwhelming urge to mentally review past relationships.

3. **Old response:** Replaying past memories, comparing feelings for his girlfriend versus others, scanning his body for groinal responses, seeking reassurance.

4. **Letting go response**
   a. He pauses and closes his eyes.
   b. He says to himself, "I'm feeling fear and shame right now. I'm not going to solve this. I'm just going to feel it."
   c. Instead of engaging with the story, he focuses on the tightness in his chest and the heat rising in his body.
   d. He sets a ten-minute timer and breathes into the discomfort.

5. **Release:** The emotions surge, then soften. The thoughts are still there, but they don't feel like emergencies anymore. He's no longer trying to *prove* anything to OCD. He's learning to let it pass.

POCD Example: "What if I'm a danger to children?"

1. **Trigger:** Stephanie sees a child at the grocery store and thinks, "What if I looked too long? What if I secretly want to harm a child?"

2. **Emotional reaction:** Intense shame, disgust, and panic.

3. **Old response:** Mentally reviewing the situation, avoiding eye contact, ruminating for hours, compulsively Googling "POCD stories" for reassurance.

4. **Letting go response:**

   a. She recognizes the urge to mentally rewind.

   b. Instead of engaging, she silently says, "This shame is here. I'm not going to argue with it. I'm going to feel it."

   c. She sits in the car, hand on her chest, and breathes through the tension in her gut.

   d. The thought feels sticky, but she doesn't follow it. She lets the emotion rise, peak, and pass.

5. **Release:** After weeks of practicing this daily, Stephanie notices a shift. The thoughts still come, but they aren't controlling her anymore. She doesn't need to prove her innocence. She just needs to allow the emotion to be felt and pass on its own.

Make the Commitment

Dr. Hawkins encourages us to make a steadfast commitment that no matter what is going on in life, we continue to surrender negative feelings as they arise.

Not someday. Not when we "have time." But as a way of being.

Here's what that means:

- When fear arises, we feel it.
- When guilt shows up, we acknowledge it.

- When shame, anger, sadness, or doubt bubble up, we don't suppress them. We welcome them.
- We make space for the feeling, and we let it pass on its own time.

This is what it means to live a surrendered life. Not a life without struggle but a life where we're no longer fighting the emotional reality of our inner world.

Letting go becomes our foundation. The more we practice it, the more peace we uncover beneath the noise.

Formal End-of-Day Letting Go Practice

One powerful way to integrate the letting go technique is to set aside time at the end of your day to process emotions that may have gotten trapped or suppressed.

Here's how it works:

1. Find a quiet space. Sit or lie down comfortably.
2. Set a timer for ten to fifteen minutes.
3. Bring to mind an emotion or topic you felt during the day—fear, guilt, sadness, anger, pride.
4. Ask yourself the letting go questions:
   a. What am I feeling right now?
   b. Could I allow myself to feel this feeling?
   c. Could I welcome it in?
   d. Could I drop the resistance to feeling it?
   e. Could I let it go?
   f. Would I let it go?
   g. When?

Let the emotion rise. Don't analyze it. Don't fix it.

This practice can also be a powerful way to process past traumas or emotional wounds. We're not reliving the trauma, but we are creating space for the unprocessed feelings to rise and release.

The more we practice, the more we clear, and the more peace we create.

> ## Key Takeaway
>
> The thought isn't the problem. It's the emotion underneath that needs to be acknowledged, felt, and released.
>
> Letting go gives that emotion space to move, so we can too.

PART 6

OPTIMIZING YOUR BRAIN AND BODY

25

WHY LIFESTYLE DESIGN MATTERS

*If we want a regulated mind, we need
to support a regulated body.*

When I first started working through OCD recovery, I focused almost entirely on the thoughts. I thought if I could just master ERP, I'd finally be free. But something was still off. I was doing exposures, using the four core responses, and sitting with uncertainty, but I still felt constantly dysregulated. Wired. Exhausted. Foggy. On edge.

That's when I realized I couldn't fully recover from OCD if other areas of my life were out of balance.

The Brain-Body Loop

OCD isn't just in our head; it's also in our nervous system.

When we're underslept, underfed, dehydrated, overstimulated, or inflamed, our brains are more reactive. Here's what that means:

- Triggers hit harder.

- Anxiety spikes faster.
- Compulsions feel more urgent.
- Recovery feels way harder.

You might be doing all the right things with ERP, but if your brain is living in a constant fight-or-flight state because of your lifestyle, it's going to keep signaling "danger," even when there is none.

This is why lifestyle design matters.

A Brain-Health-Centric Lifestyle

Living a brain-health-centric lifestyle is about building a daily rhythm that supports nervous system health and mental clarity. It means paying attention to the basics that most of us are never taught to prioritize:

- Sleep
- Nutrition
- Movement
- Mindfulness and meditation
- Supplements (in some cases)
- How we use our phone
- How much stimulation we take in
- Who we spend time with
- How we spend our time

These aren't nice-to-haves. They're core parts of the recovery journey.

OCD Feeds on Dysregulation

Let me be clear: OCD *loves* a dysregulated body.

He feeds on these:

- Sleep deprivation

- Blood sugar crashes
- Chronic stress
- Digital overload
- Caffeine overload
- Loneliness

These things don't cause OCD, but they absolutely turn the volume up. They keep us in survival mode, where compulsions feel necessary just to make it through the day. Recovery becomes so much more sustainable when we support the brain biologically, not just behaviorally.

Key Takeaway

You can't outthink a dysregulated body.

When we support our brain with consistent sleep, blood sugar balance, movement, hydration, nature, meditation, and mindful inputs, we make it easier to do the work OCD recovery requires.

We'll discuss these tools more in the coming chapters.

26

SLEEP

We can't beat OCD when
we're running on fumes.

If there's one thing I wish someone had told me earlier in my recovery, it's this: Sleep is not optional.

Not if we want our brain to function. Not if we want to lower anxiety. Not if we want to have even a sliver of mental clarity to practice ERP, apply mindset tools, or resist compulsions.

We treat sleep like a luxury, but it's a requirement for healing.

Why Sleep Matters So Much for OCD

When we're sleep-deprived, the brain goes into threat mode. The amygdala (our fear center) becomes overactive. The prefrontal cortex (rational thinking, impulse control) shuts down. Here's what that can create:

- More intrusive thoughts
- More emotional reactivity
- More compulsions

- More intensity in how we experience thoughts and feelings

Lack of sleep doesn't just make us tired. It makes us more vulnerable to OCD's lies.

Poor Sleep = More OCD

Here's how the cycle often works:

1. OCD flares up, so intrusive thoughts keep us anxious or ruminating at night.
2. We don't sleep well, so our baseline anxiety increases.
3. Our brain is foggy, so we're more likely to compulse to get relief.
4. Compulsions spike our stress, so sleep gets worse again.

It's a vicious loop.

The good news is that even small improvements to our sleep can break this cycle and lower our reactivity dramatically.

How Much Sleep Do We Really Need?

According to the American Academy of Sleep Medicine, the Sleep Research Society,[10] and the National Sleep Foundation,[11] the ideal amount of sleep for adults is seven to nine hours per night. Less than that on a regular basis can increase anxiety, worsen intrusive thoughts, and make recovery harder.

I've personally noticed that my ideal amount of sleep is between eight and nine hours each night. Anything under seven and OCD tends to be more prevalent the next day.

OCD and Sleep Anxiety

OCD can latch on to the act of sleep itself. The fear of *not* falling asleep can become its own obsession. We get sticky thoughts like "What if I don't fall asleep and tomorrow is ruined?" and "I'll feel awful unless I fall asleep right now."

These pressures create more anxiety, which ironically makes it even harder to fall asleep.

Not to worry, though. We can apply the tools we learned about in earlier chapters. Acceptance, indifference, uncertainty, agreement, and the letting go technique are powerful allies at bedtime. Instead of fighting to fall asleep, try saying this: "Maybe I will fall asleep, maybe I won't. I'll rest either way."

Better Sleep Through ERP

If intrusive thoughts are keeping you up at night, you're not alone. Once you start doing ERP consistently, your brain learns that these thoughts aren't emergencies. Over time, the thoughts will become less frequent, less intense, and less sticky. That makes it easier to fall asleep without needing to fight or figure out every thought before bed.

Sleep Is a Biological Process—Not a Performance

As noted above, one of the biggest traps is trying to *force* sleep. The more we pressure ourselves, the more alert our brain becomes. Just like we can't force ourselves to fall in love or laugh genuinely at a joke, we can't *force* ourselves into sleep. It's a biological process that happens on its own time when our brain is ready. That said, there are steps we can take to help ourselves sleep more easily.

Keys to Better Sleep

These are the basic pillars we focus on:

1. Protect Your Wind-Down Window

- Start winding down sixty to ninety minutes before bed.
- Don't look at emails, scroll, or engage in triggering conversations.
- Keep lights dim, and use blue-light blockers if needed.
- Do something slow: stretching, journaling, reading, meditation.

2. Go to Bed at the Same Time Every Night

Our brain thrives on rhythm. A consistent bedtime helps regulate our circadian clock and reduce cortisol spikes at night. This isn't about perfection, though. Being relatively consistent is good enough.

3. Keep Your Bedroom Cool, Dark, and Screen-Free

Your brain needs external cues that it's time to rest. Use blackout curtains, lower the temp, and charge your phone in another room if you can.

4. Avoid Stimulants in the Afternoon

Caffeine stays in our system for up to ten hours. If you're struggling with racing thoughts or nighttime anxiety, consider cutting off caffeine by noon.

5. Don't Try to Sleep—Try to Rest

If you can't fall asleep, get out of bed. Sit somewhere else and do something calming. Don't pressure yourself to force sleep. The more we chase sleep, the more elusive it becomes.

Nighttime Meditation

Calming the nervous system before bed can make a huge difference. Nighttime meditations help us create the internal safety needed to let go and rest.

Natural Tools for Sleep

If you're struggling to physically settle, these natural supplements may help:

- **L-theanine:** This helps relax the nervous system without making you drowsy.
- **Magnesium glycinate:** This supports sleep and anxiety regulation.
- **Magnesium taurate:** This regulates a pounding heart.

Environmental Tools That Make a Big Difference

Don't underestimate the power of your sleep environment. If you're sensitive to sound or light, these two small tools can help dramatically:

- **Earplugs:** These block out distracting or jarring noise.
- **Eye mask:** This keeps light from interfering with melatonin production.

I personally use both, and they've significantly improved the quality of my sleep.

A Note on Alcohol and Cannabis

It's common to reach for a glass of wine or a cannabis gummy to help wind down. And yes—these substances can make us feel sleepy or relaxed in the moment.

Here's the catch: According to research, both alcohol[12] and cannabis[13] inhibit REM sleep, which is one of the most important stages for emotional regulation, memory processing, and overall brain recovery.

Here's what less REM means:

- Higher baseline anxiety the next day
- Less emotional resilience
- Increased OCD reactivity

I'm not saying you can never indulge. That's a values-based choice, and it's personal for each of us. But I am suggesting we stay mindful. If you notice OCD hits harder the morning after you drink alcohol or use cannabis, it's not your imagination. These substances might help you *fall* asleep, but they'll likely affect the *quality* of your sleep, and that absolutely impacts your recovery.

Key Takeaway

Sleep is not about perfection; it's about creating the right conditions for rest. If OCD turns sleep into another obsession, respond with acceptance, indifference, and letting go. Your job is to rest, not perform. Sleep will naturally happen on its own time.

EXERCISE

Movement isn't just good for the body;
it's medicine for our mind.

When we're struggling with OCD, anxiety, or low mood, there's one tool that can get overlooked: moving our body. We often treat exercise as a way to change how we look. In the context of OCD recovery, it's about how we *feel* mentally, emotionally, and neurologically. Exercise isn't just about fitness. It's about regulation.

Why Exercise Helps with OCD

When we move our body, especially in sustained aerobic activity, it helps us do the following:

- Regulate our nervous system
- Reduce baseline anxiety levels
- Increase feel-good brain chemicals (like serotonin, dopamine, and endorphins)[14]
- Improve focus, clarity, and mood

- Improve our sleep quality (which we now know is essential for recovery)

This isn't woo-woo; it's neuroscience. Movement helps shift our body out of fight-or-flight mode and into a more calm, balanced, responsive state.

The more regulated we are, the easier it becomes to face fears, resist compulsions, and do the hard work of recovery.

It Doesn't Have to Be Perfect

One of the most common traps we OCDers can fall into is perfectionism around exercise, which, ironically, is often fueled by OCD itself. The discomfort of not doing it "right" or "enough" can become so overwhelming that we end up doing nothing at all.

The real problem is that when OCD keeps us frozen in perfectionism, we end up dropping movement entirely. And when we drop a coping strategy, our anxiety builds.

The solution? Treat exercise like exposure work. Do it imperfectly on purpose. Let yourself show up messy, disorganized, or inconsistent. Practice letting go of needing to do it perfectly.

You don't need a perfect routine. You don't need to hit the gym for hours a day (even if your brain tells you so). You just need to move your body consistently in a way that feels sustainable.

Start with these ideas:

- A ten-minute walk in the morning
- Dancing to music in your kitchen
- A short yoga or mobility video on YouTube
- Jumping jacks in your living room
- A fifteen- to twenty-minute gym session

What matters most is that you're showing up gently and consistently. That's the win.

My Personal Approach to Exercise

Even now, years into my recovery journey, I still don't think about exercise in terms of how I look. I think about how it makes me feel. For me, movement is a nervous system regulation tool. That's it.

If I go a few days without moving my body, just lying around or out of rhythm, I can feel the difference. The anxious energy builds. My body feels tense and my thoughts get louder.

Even a short workout or walk outside in nature can start to release that pressure. It doesn't have to be intense. It just has to be consistent.

That's why movement remains a nonnegotiable for me. It helps keep my mind grounded and my recovery on track.

Types of Movement to Explore

There's no one-size-fits-all approach to exercise. Everyone's body—and nervous system—is different. The key is to find what works for *you*.

Here are some types of movement you might consider:

- **Walking or hiking:** low impact, calming, easy to start (preferably in nature)
- **Strength training:** builds resilience, improves confidence, helps release emotions like anger
- **Running:** boosts endorphins, clears the mind, regulates anxiety
- **Yoga:** combines movement and mindfulness, stimulates the vagus nerve
- **Cycling:** rhythmic, grounding
- **Swimming:** low impact, deeply regulating
- **Dancing:** expressive, energizing
- **Pilates or mobility work:** helps connect with your body gently

- **Team or group sports:** adds a social element that supports mood

You don't have to love it; you just need to feel some benefit from it. Movement doesn't have to be intense or complicated. It just has to be yours.

Movement = Momentum

The more we move, the more momentum we build. Not just physically, but mentally.

You might start your day feeling foggy or anxious, but after a short walk, you're more clear. You might be stuck in a spiral, but after a workout, the thoughts feel less loud.

Movement gets us out of our heads and back into our bodies.

How I Incorporate Movement into My Life

To this day, movement is a foundational part of how I support my nervous system. Here's how I work it into my life:

- I start each morning with ten to fifteen minutes of meditation followed by a walk outside. This helps clear my head and regulate my body before the day begins.
- I try to get in a run, boxing session, or lifting session three to four times a week. This is not to chase a physique goal but to release tension and stay grounded.
- Most weekdays, I finish the day with a nature walk with my wife, either on the beach or in a nearby preserve. It's become one of the most meaningful and calming rituals in my routine.

None of this is about being perfect. I genuinely enjoy these habits and look forward to them. My hope is that you'll find forms of movement that feel true to you. Exercise doesn't "cure" OCD on its own. ERP and resisting compulsions are still the foundation of recovery. But exercise supports recovery by strengthening your brain and body—helping you regulate stress, tolerate discomfort, and show up more consistently for the actual OCD work.

Key Takeaway

You don't need a perfect fitness plan. You need consistency.

Move your body to shift your brain. Even ten minutes a day can make OCD recovery more manageable.

Call to Action

Get Moving

Take two minutes right now and choose one form of movement you want to try—whether it's a walk, a light workout, or dancing in your kitchen. Then commit to giving it a shot tomorrow—just start, even if it's not perfect.

28

MEDITATION AND MINDFULNESS

I started meditating in 2015, long before I had language for what I was really struggling with. At the time, my mind was chaotic with an endless stream of intrusive thoughts, fear, doubt, and confusion. I hadn't been formally diagnosed with OCD yet, but I knew something was deeply off.

That's when I stumbled upon Andy Puddicombe and his guided meditations. His voice, his pacing, and the simplicity of his approach helped cut through the noise in my brain. Andy was also the first to introduce me to the concept that all thoughts are like passing clouds in the sky—meant to be observed, not clung to. That idea gave me hope.

At the time, every thought felt sticky. I felt stuck. This metaphor showed me there was another way to relate to my mind. It didn't cure the OCD, but it gave me moments of calm when nothing else could. Those meditations, quite literally, saved me early in my journey.

They've stuck with me ever since. Over the years, meditation has become a staple in my daily life. Today, I've logged over forty thousand minutes of meditation, and I can confidently say that outside of ERP, the four core responses, and the letting go technique, meditation is the single most important tool I've used to manage OCD.

Meditation is not magic. It's not a quick fix. But it helps us build the muscle we need to sit with discomfort, observe our thoughts, and stop reacting to everything OCD throws our way.

What Meditation Does for the Brain

We often think meditation is just about "clearing the mind." But what it's really doing is changing our brain's operating system.

Studies show that consistent meditation does the following:

- Reduces the size and reactivity of the amygdala (our fear center)
- Strengthens the prefrontal cortex (where logic, decision-making, and impulse control live)
- Improves attention and emotional regulation
- Lower baseline anxiety and stress

For us OCDers, meditation has also been shown to reduce symptom severity, increase distress tolerance, and create more space between thought and compulsion.

It's like going to the gym, but for our brain.[15]

Brain Waves and Mindfulness

Our brains operate on different frequencies depending on what we're doing. Here's a breakdown:

- **Gamma:** high-level cognitive functioning, deep insight
- **Beta:** normal waking consciousness, thinking, analyzing (where OCD thrives)
- **Alpha:** calm, restful awareness (what meditation helps us achieve)
- **Theta:** deep relaxation, light sleep, creativity
- **Delta:** deep sleep

Meditation helps shift us out of beta and into alpha, theta, and sometimes even gamma—the states where the nervous system calms down, the body relaxes, and healing happens.

For OCDers, this is crucial. It gives our mind and body a chance to reset without needing compulsions to create relief.[16]

Debunking Myths About Meditation

Let's clear something up: Meditation is not about emptying our mind of thoughts. We're not trying to stop thinking or block thoughts. The harder we try not to think, the more thoughts we bring on.

Meditation also isn't the same as prayer, and it doesn't have to be tied to any religious or spiritual belief. You don't have to subscribe to any tradition to practice meditation.

Meditation trains OCDers to sit with our thoughts and feelings, noticing when our mind has wandered and then gently bringing ourselves back to the present moment over and over again.

If you're getting distracted a hundred times, you're doing it right. The practice is in noticing you've wandered and bringing your attention back to your breath.

How to Approach Meditation

Starting a meditation practice doesn't have to be complicated. You don't need to sit for hours or turn off all your thoughts. You just need a few minutes and a willingness to show up for yourself.

Here are a few tips to get started:

- **Use a guide.** Especially early on, guided meditations are incredibly helpful. They give your mind an anchor and teach you how to come back to the present moment. You can find options with platforms like Headspace or Insight Timer.
- **Keep it short.** Five to ten minutes is plenty when you're getting started. You can build over time, but what matters most is consistency, not duration.
- **Find a quiet space.** Choose a place where you can sit without distraction. You don't need complete silence, just fewer interruptions.
- **Set a timer.** Even a few minutes of dedicated practice makes a difference.
- **Don't aim for perfection.** Your mind will wander. You'll forget you're meditating. That's normal. The practice is in returning to your breath.

Meditation Is Training for Rumination Freedom

One of the reasons meditation is so powerful in OCD recovery is because it helps us work with one of the most common compulsions of all: **rumination**.

As you've already learned, rumination is the mental ritual of analyzing, debating, reviewing, and trying to "figure it out" until we feel relief. And because it happens quietly in our head, it can be hard to catch. It can even feel like we're being responsible or "working through" something. But in reality, rumination is one of the main ways OCD keeps itself alive.

This is where meditation becomes more than just a relaxation tool. Meditation is practice for our brain. It trains us to:

- notice a thought,
- label it as a thought,
- and gently redirect our attention back to the present

That exact process is one of the core skills of recovery.

When OCD throws a scary thought at us, we don't need to solve it—we need to recognize what's happening and stop feeding it. Meditation helps us build this skill in a calm, controlled environment. It teaches us to relate to thoughts differently—without urgency, without panic, and without needing to "complete" the thought.

A Simple Example

Let's say you're meditating and focusing on your breathing. Then a thought pops up: "What if I'm a bad person?"

In the past, you might have automatically started spiraling: "Why did I think that?" "Does that mean something?" "Let me prove it isn't true."

But in meditation, we practice a new response. You simply notice it and label it: "Thought." Or "OCD thought."

And then, without arguing with it or trying to make it go away, you gently return your attention back to your breath: Inhale . . . Exhale . . .

That's it.

That tiny moment—noticing, labeling, and returning—is the skill. And every rep makes it easier to do the same thing in real life when OCD shows up loudly.

So when you're meditating and your mind wanders, you're not failing. That moment is the whole point. Every time you catch yourself drifting into a mental story and gently return to the breath, the body, or the present moment, you're practicing. You're learning that you don't have to engage with every thought.

The goal isn't to clear your mind or feel peaceful 100 percent of the time. The goal is to train your brain to stop treating thoughts like threats—and start treating them like what they really are: mental noise that you don't have to obey.

Key Takeaway

Meditation isn't about controlling your thoughts. It's about learning to watch them without fear.

Over time, it rewires your brain to feel safe inside your body again. In OCD recovery, that's one of the most powerful gifts you can give yourself.

29

NATURE AND NERVOUS SYSTEM REGULATION

*Sometimes the best way to quiet
the mind is to step outside.*

When I think about what's helped me most on this recovery journey, especially when my nervous system has felt fried, it's not always a tool or a technique. Sometimes, it's as simple as stepping outside.

Spending time in nature has been one of the most regulating, healing practices in my life. It doesn't have to be dramatic. It could be a walk by the beach, sitting under a tree, or walking through a quiet neighborhood with my wife at sunset.

These moments remind me I'm not just my thoughts. There is a bigger life outside of the four walls of my home, despite what fear OCD keeps trying to sell me.

What Nature Does to the Brain

Science backs up what many of us have felt intuitively for years, which is that nature is medicine for the mind.

Time spent in natural environments has been shown to do the following:

- Lower cortisol (our stress hormone)
- Reduce heart rate and blood pressure
- Improve mood and emotional regulation
- Quiet the default mode network (the part of our brain linked to rumination)
- Increase vagal tone (linked to better resilience and nervous system recovery)

Put simply, nature helps our nervous system reset. As shown in research from the National Academy of Sciences, when our nervous system feels safer, it becomes easier to respond to OCD with clarity instead of panic.[17]

Designed for the Outdoors

Evolutionarily, we're not meant to live indoors, hunched over screens, disconnected from natural rhythms. For thousands of years, humans lived in tune with nature walking, hunting, gathering, and resting under the stars.

In his book *Lost Connections*, author Johann Hari highlights how much of our mental health crisis is rooted in disconnection from meaning, from community, and from nature itself.[18] One of the most overlooked truths? We heal better when we're in environments we were actually designed for.

Reconnecting with nature, even in small ways, can help rewire a nervous system that's spent too long in survival mode.

It Doesn't Have to Be Complicated

We don't need a cabin in the woods or a silent retreat to feel the benefits of nature, although those are okay too.

Try these ideas:

- Walking through a tree-lined street for ten minutes
- Sitting on your porch and noticing the wind or clouds
- Walking along a beach boardwalk or through a nature preserve
- Leaving your phone at home and walking mindfully around the block
- Taking a more strenuous hike (depending on what's appropriate for you)

The point isn't to do nature perfectly. The point is to let your body catch a break from overstimulation.

My Personal Nature Rituals

Every weekday, my wife and I end our day with a nature walk. Sometimes it's by the beach, and other times it's through a local preserve. It's become a ritual that helps us downshift out of work mode and reconnect with our bodies. No phone. No work talk. Just attempting to be present.

These small moments help build space in my brain to realize my thoughts aren't as important as I sometimes think they are. It also helps my nervous system calm down, which makes resting in the evening and falling asleep easier. The chain of connections makes me feel better equipped to handle what OCD throws at me.

Nature helps us come back into balance. It's not a luxury—it's part of recovery. It literally alters our physiology. Please do not ignore this chapter. Getting into nature won't cure OCD, but it will significantly improve rumination and anxiety when done consistently.

Key Takeaway

We're not designed to live in front of screens, under fluorescent lights, and inside our heads 24/7.

30

SUPPLEMENTS

*You can't supplement your way out
of OCD, but the right ones can
support the process.*

Supplements aren't a cure for OCD, and they shouldn't be your first line of defense. When used *alongside* tools like ERP, the letting go technique, meditation, nutrition, medication, and movement, they can absolutely support brain and nervous system health.

Think of them like this: Supplements don't replace the work. They help you recover in a body that's more regulated and resilient.

Everyone's body is different, so always consult a health care provider, but here are some of the most researched and commonly used supplements in the OCD recovery community.

L-Theanine[19]

- **What it does:** This amino acid found in green tea promotes calm without sedation.
- **Why it helps:** It supports alpha brain wave production, associated with calm alertness.
- **How to use it:** Take it in capsule or powder form. Many use 100 mg to 200 mg before bed or during high-stress periods.
- **How I use it:** I take this daily.

GABA

- **What it does:** This calming neurotransmitter can help reduce overexcitability in the brain.
- **Why it helps:** It supports the nervous system and can ease physical tension.
- **How to use it:** Take it as a capsule or lozenge. It is often used before sleep or during anxious spikes.
- **How I use it:** I take this as needed.

Mood Probiotic[20]

- **What it does:** It targets the gut-brain axis and supports serotonin production.
- **Why it helps:** A healthy gut supports a healthy mood; some strains are designed specifically for anxiety or depression.
- **How to use it:** Take it daily. Look for multistrain formulas that include lactobacillus and bifidobacterium.
- **How I use it:** I cycle on and off this.

Fish Oil (Omega-3s)[21]

- **What it does:** It supports cognitive function and reduces inflammation.
- **Why it helps:** It may support mood and reduce symptoms of anxiety and depression.
- **How to use it:** Take 1,000 mg to 2,000 mg daily; choose high-quality, purified brands.

B12

- **What it does:** It supports energy, brain function, and nervous system health.
- **Why it helps:** B12 deficiency can worsen anxiety and mental fatigue.
- **How to use it:** It can be taken sublingually, in a capsule, or via injection if you're deficient.

B Complex

- **What it does:** This blend of B vitamins works to support energy production, brain function, and stress resilience.
- **Why it helps:** B vitamins (especially B6, B9, and B12) are involved in neurotransmitter regulation and may reduce symptoms of anxiety and low mood.
- **How to use it:** This is often taken in the morning with food. Choose a high-quality, activated formula.
- **How I use it:** I take this daily, but cycle on and off.

Vitamin D3[22]

- **What it does:** It regulates mood and immune function.

- **Why it helps:** Many with OCD and anxiety are deficient in D3, especially in low-sunlight areas.
- **How to use it:** Take 1,000 IU to 4,000 IU a day; test your levels before supplementing.
- **How I use it:** I take this as needed.

Ashwagandha

- **What it does:** This adaptogen supports the body's stress response.
- **Why it helps:** It may reduce cortisol and promote calm focus.
- **How to use it:** Take it in capsule or powder form. This is often used at night or during stressful seasons.
- **How I use it:** I take this as needed.

Magnesium (Glycinate, Threonate, Citrate, Taurate)

As discussed earlier, there are several forms of magnesium, and each has its own strengths:

- **Magnesium glycinate:** Known for its calming effects, this is great for anxiety and sleep support. It's also gentle on the stomach.
- **Magnesium threonate:** This crosses the blood-brain barrier and may support cognitive function and mental clarity.
- **Magnesium citrate:** This helps with digestion and regularity. It's best taken earlier in the day if used for this purpose.
- **Magnesium taurate:** This combines magnesium with taurine to support both cardiovascular and nervous system health. It may be helpful for calming the body and reducing anxiety-related symptoms like heart palpitations.

You don't need to take all of these forms of magnesium. Many people benefit from choosing the one that aligns best with their specific need—whether that's sleep, anxiety, digestion, or heart and nervous system balance.

Turmeric (Curcumin)

- **What it does:** This has anti-inflammatory and antioxidant properties.
- **Why it helps:** Chronic inflammation can worsen mental health symptoms.
- **How to use it:** Take capsules or add it to food with black pepper for absorption.

Golden Milk (Turmeric Latte)

- **What it does:** This warm turmeric-based drink that supports inflammation reduction and keeping the nervous system calm.
- **Why it helps:** Turmeric (curcumin) has anti-inflammatory properties, and this drink can become a calming ritual for the body and brain.
- **How to use it:** You can drink it in the morning or evening. Many people make it with warm milk (or almond/oat milk), turmeric, cinnamon, ginger, and a pinch of black pepper for absorption.
- **How I use it:** I started drinking golden milk and it made a noticeable difference for me—my chronic headaches and chest pain went away, and the pounding feeling in my heart I used to get at night dramatically reduced. I drink two a day, one in the morning and one at night.

Lemon Balm

- **What it does:** This calming herb has been used for centuries to support mood.

- **Why it helps:** It can reduce anxiety and support sleep.
- **How to use it:** It's often found in teas, tinctures, or capsules.

Stress Tea

- **What it does:** Herbal blends can help the body wind down.
- **Why it helps:** Noncaffeinated herbs like chamomile, lavender, and passionflower promote relaxation.
- **How to use it:** Drink it in the evening as part of your wind-down routine.

NAC (N-Acetyl Cysteine)[23]

- **What it does:** This is a precursor to glutathione, the body's master antioxidant.
- **Why it helps:** Some studies suggest NAC may help reduce OCD symptoms by modulating glutamate levels in the brain.
- **How to use it:** Common dosage ranges from 600 mg to 2,400 mg a day, often in divided doses; always consult with a health care provider first.

Inositol[24]

- **What it does:** This natural sugar alcohol and component of cell membranes affects serotonin activity in the brain.
- **Why it helps:** Clinical research shows inositol, especially in higher doses (12 g to 18 g a day), may reduce OCD symptoms and improve emotional regulation.
- **How to use it:** It's typically taken in powder form, mixed into water or juice. Start slow and increase under supervision to avoid GI side effects.

Saffron

- **What it does:** Saffron is a spice derived from the *Crocus sativus* flower, traditionally used for mood support and cognitive health.
- **Why it helps:** Research suggests saffron may help improve mood, reduce symptoms of depression and anxiety, and support overall emotional well-being, potentially making OCD recovery work more manageable.
- **How to use it:** Common dosage in studies ranges from 15 mg to 30 mg daily, usually split into two doses. Always consult with a healthcare provider about dosage.

A Note Before You Supplement

Before adding any supplements to your routine, always consult with your doctor or a licensed health care provider.

Some supplements may interact with medications or other conditions. What works well for one person may not be safe or helpful for another. Always consider where you are purchasing your supplements from to ensure that only the highest quality ingredients are being used.

Example Supplement Schedule

This is a general schedule based on what many clients find supportive—but it's not a prescription. Modify it based on your body's needs and what your provider recommends.

Morning

- Vitamin D3
- B12 or B complex

- Fish oil
- Mood probiotic

Afternoon (If Needed)

- NAC
- Ashwagandha (if taken twice a day)

Evening

- L-theanine
- Magnesium glycinate or threonate
- GABA (as needed)
- Stress tea or lemon balm

You Don't Need Everything

It's easy to feel like you need to take every supplement listed here, but that's not the goal. Start small. Test one addition at a time and notice how your body responds.

Everyone's system is different. The goal is to find the few supplements that support *your* recovery—it's not to build a pharmacy in your kitchen.

A Thought on Testosterone (for Men)

Some emerging research suggests that low testosterone levels may contribute to increased anxiety, low mood, and even obsessive-compulsive symptoms in men. While testosterone isn't a "cure" for OCD, supporting your overall hormonal health could help regulate your nervous system and improve energy, motivation, and mental clarity.

I want to share something personal: A few years back, I had my blood work done and discovered that my testosterone levels were low. Around the same time, a client I was working with did the same and received similar results.

We both started supplementing and making lifestyle changes to naturally support testosterone production—prioritizing sleep, reducing stimulant use, doing strength training, and using targeted supplementation under medical guidance.[25]

The difference was noticeable:

- Increased energy
- Decreased fatigue
- More stable mood
- Improved quality of thoughts

I fully recognize that this is anecdotal, and I'm not saying testosterone is the missing link for everyone. But if you feel chronically depleted—especially as a man—it's something to consider and talk to your doctor about. It's not about hacking your hormones; it's about making sure your system is supported so you can show up for the deeper work of recovery.

But remember, testosterone therapy or supplementation should *always* be done under the guidance of a licensed medical professional.

A Note on Estrogen and Hormonal Health (for Women)

Just like testosterone plays a key role in men's emotional regulation, estrogen plays a massive role for women.

Estrogen helps regulate the following[26]:

- Stress responses via the HPA axis
- Serotonin and dopamine (mood-related neurotransmitters)

- Memory, focus, and verbal learning

When estrogen levels drop—whether from menstrual cycles, postpartum shifts, perimenopause, or menopause—many women experience an increase in anxiety, intrusive thoughts, and brain fog.

Important Note About Estrogen and OCD

Many women find their OCD symptoms spike during their menstrual cycle, especially in the week leading up to their period. This is due to natural hormonal shifts, and it's not a sign that you're going backward. It's a real, biological sensitivity. Just knowing this can help you meet those days with more self-compassion and awareness.

If you're noticing worsening symptoms around hormonal changes, talk to your doctor or a functional medicine provider. There may be safe, natural ways to support hormonal balance, from nutrition and stress management to supplements and (in some cases) hormone therapy.

I've worked with clients who began supporting their hormone health and noticed significant shifts in these areas:

- Energy
- Mood
- Mental clarity
- Most importantly, their ability to apply the tools in this book

It's not a silver bullet, but it's a piece of the puzzle worth paying attention to. Always consult a licensed medical professional before starting any hormonal or supplement regimen.

Get the Full Picture

Before diving into any supplement routine, I highly recommend getting your blood work done and reviewed by a licensed medical provider or a functional medicine doctor. Everyone's body is different. A trained professional can help you identify any deficiencies, hormonal imbalances, or nutritional gaps, and they can work with you to create a supplement plan that's safe, effective, and personalized for your recovery.

Key Takeaway

Supplements aren't a magic pill, and we shouldn't look at them as a "cure." But they can make our recovery tools more effective and support your brain in becoming more balanced so that you can do the work that leads to freedom.

31

MEDICATION

A TOOL, NOT A SHORTCUT

*There's no shame in needing support.
Just don't forget the work that actually
rewires your brain.*

Let me start by being crystal clear: For many years, I never took medication for OCD, but I've always believed there should be no stigma attached to it. Medication can be a helpful support tool in OCD recovery. It's not a failure, it's not cheating, and it doesn't mean you're weak.

And I also want to share an update: I'm currently taking 50 mg of Zoloft, and it's been genuinely helpful for me. It hasn't "cured" me, but it has lowered the volume enough to give me more space to use the tools consistently and feel more like myself again.

Medication can be incredibly helpful—and for some people, it may even be enough. But for many people, the best long-term results come from combining medication with the tools and strategies you've been learning throughout this book. Medication can calm the nervous system and lower the intensity, but the tools—ERP, acceptance, letting go—are what teach your brain a new way to respond.

I've had conversations with people from all over the world who are on medication for OCD. And the story is often the same: "It helped. It gave me a little space. But the tools—ERP, acceptance, letting go—that's what truly changed my life."

So, if you're considering medication, here's what you need to know.

How Medication Works for OCD

Most of the medications used to treat OCD fall under a class called *selective serotonin reuptake inhibitors (SSRIs)*. These medications work by increasing serotonin activity in the brain, which is believed to help reduce obsessive thoughts and compulsive urges.

In some cases, a class called *serotonin-norepinephrine reuptake inhibitors (SNRIs)* might be prescribed, or perhaps *tricyclic antidepressants (TCAs)*—especially if SSRIs haven't worked or aren't well tolerated.

Some individuals also benefit from low-dose antipsychotics added as augmenting agents, but this is typically reserved for more severe or treatment-resistant cases and always managed under close medical supervision.

Common Medications Prescribed for OCD

- **SSRIs (first-line treatment):**
  - Fluoxetine (Prozac)
  - Fluvoxamine (Luvox)

- ◦ Sertraline (Zoloft)
- ◦ Paroxetine (Paxil)
- ◦ Citalopram (Celexa)
- ◦ Escitalopram (Lexapro)
- **TCA (often used when SSRIs don't work):**
  - ◦ Clomipramine (Anafranil)—one of the oldest and most researched medications for OCD
- **Other augmenting options (used alongside an SSRI):**
  - ◦ Aripiprazole (Abilify)
  - ◦ Risperidone (Risperdal)
  - ◦ Low-dose antipsychotics (only under psychiatric supervision)

A Word of Caution

I am not a licensed psychiatrist or medical professional. Nothing in this chapter should be taken as medical advice.

If you're considering medication, you need to consult with a licensed psychiatrist who understands OCD. They'll help you weigh the pros and cons, evaluate your history, and monitor your progress. Medication should always be personalized and carefully supervised.

What I've Learned from the Community

As I emphasized at the start of this chapter, I've heard a common theme again and again in the course of my work: "The meds helped reduce the noise, but it was the mindset shifts, the exposures, and the acceptance work that gave me my life back."

If you do take medication, let it support your work—not replace it. Use it to help create a little space between you and ODC. Then use that space to dive into the tools that rewire your brain for good.

Key Takeaway

Medication can be a powerful support tool, but it's not a cure. The real change comes from how we respond to the thoughts, not whether we have them.

There's no shame in being on medication and getting help. Just remember that the tools in this book are still the foundation of your freedom.

32

SUBSTANCES

What we put in our body affects
what happens in our mind.

'll be honest—this chapter might challenge you, and that's okay.
It challenged me too.

My goal isn't to tell you what you can or can't do. My goal is to help you make informed, empowered choices when it comes to substances like alcohol, cannabis, caffeine, and even nicotine.

Why? Because what we consume can either support or sabotage our OCD recovery.

Alcohol and OCD[27]

Alcohol can feel like a relief in the moment. It takes the edge off. It quiets the noise. But there's a cost.

Alcohol disrupts sleep, impairs emotional regulation, and inhibits REM sleep, the stage responsible for memory consolidation and emotional recovery. It might help us fall asleep faster, but it lowers the quality of our rest. Lower-quality sleep means higher anxiety and OCD reactivity the next day.

It can also reduce our ability to use tools like ERP and letting go effectively. We're more emotionally reactive and less mentally sharp.

I'm not saying never drink. That's a values-based choice. I am saying you should pay attention to how you feel the day after drinking. Notice the patterns. OCD thrives when we're depleted.

Here's another side to it: Some people with OCD avoid alcohol entirely, not for health reasons but out of fear. Fear that they'll lose control. Fear they'll do something they can't remember or that they'll regret. Fear they'll spiral. This kind of rigid avoidance can become a compulsion in itself. So while I'm not encouraging drinking, I want to be clear that avoiding alcohol out of fear, rather than values, is something to examine.

Cannabis and OCD[28]

Like alcohol, cannabis may feel like it helps in the moment, especially with sleep or calming the mind.

But studies show it can inhibit REM sleep, alter memory and learning, and sometimes worsen anxiety and paranoia over time. For us OCDers, this can be a dangerous loop, especially if we're using cannabis to escape intrusive thoughts.

Additionally, using cannabis to numb or escape can prevent us from learning how to tolerate discomfort naturally, and that's a key skill in recovery.

Again, this isn't about judgment. It's about awareness. If cannabis is keeping you from facing your fears or if it's making your symptoms worse over time, it's worth reevaluating.

Caffeine and OCD[29]

Caffeine is one of the most widely used stimulants on the planet. For many of us with anxiety or OCD, it's a double-edged sword.

Caffeine ramps up the nervous system. It increases heart rate, heightens alertness, and, in some people, mimics the symptoms of an OCD spike—racing thoughts, restlessness, and panic. It also spikes cortisol in the body, which, if sustained for long periods of time, can lead to chronic fatigue and a decrease in testosterone for men.

If you're sensitive to caffeine or already feeling on edge, it might make OCD feel more intense. It can also interfere with sleep, which we know is foundational to recovery.

If you use caffeine, try these ideas:

- Limit it to the morning.
- Eat beforehand (don't drink it on an empty stomach).
- Choose lower-stimulant options like matcha or green tea.

Nicotine and OCD[30]

Some people use nicotine to cope with anxiety, boredom, or stress. While it can give a temporary sense of focus or relief, it's short-lived.

Nicotine spikes adrenaline and dopamine, but it often leads to a crash in mood shortly after. It also activates the sympathetic nervous system—the fight-or-flight response—which is already overactive in us OCDers.

Like other substances, it's a short-term relief that can lead to long-term dysregulation.

Values-Based Living

Let me be up front with you: I still drink alcohol from time to time. My wife and I might split a bottle of wine on a weekend, and I enjoy it because I get to spend intentional time with her. Caffeine? It was a staple in my life for over a decade. While I've drastically reduced how much I consume, and I don't drink it on an empty stomach, I still use it occasionally when I feel it supports me.

This isn't about perfection. It's about being honest with yourself about your values, your goals, and how your behaviors impact your recovery. Values-based living means making intentional choices based on what matters most to you, not what OCD tells you to fear or avoid.

The Bottom Line

I'm not here to tell you to cut out everything. I am here to encourage curiosity and compassionate experimentation.

Ask yourself these questions:

- "Is this substance helping me feel more resilient or more reactive?"
- "Am I using this to cope with feelings I could learn to tolerate naturally?"
- "How do I feel the next day—mentally, emotionally, and physically?"

You deserve a recovery that's supported—not sabotaged—by what you put in your body.

Key Takeaway

Substances aren't inherently bad, but they do have an impact. Approach them with awareness. Use your body's feedback as your guide.

33

DIGITAL HYGIENE AND DOPAMINE

*If your brain always needs a hit,
it won't know how to sit.*

We live in a world designed to keep our brains overstimulated. Between constant notifications, endless scrolling, and apps engineered to hijack our attention, most of us are *wired but tired*—anxious, distracted, and burned out without knowing why.

For OCDers especially, this matters. A brain that's overstimulated is a brain that's more reactive. And a reactive brain is way more likely to fall into the OCD cycle.

The Dopamine Problem

Our digital devices are dopamine machines. Every ping, swipe, and scroll gives us a little burst of feel-good chemical that keeps us coming back.

But over time, that constant dopamine drip trains our brain to expect stimulation 24/7. When we don't get it, we feel anxious, restless, and even irritable. That discomfort makes intrusive thoughts feel louder, more threatening, and harder to sit with.

It's not a character flaw; it's neuroscience. It means part of recovery is giving our brain a break from constant dopamine and a chance to reset.

What Overstimulation Looks Like

I've noticed in my own life that when I'm feeling stressed or overwhelmed by work or my thoughts, I tend to reach for my phone more often. I'll start doomscrolling, trying to escape from the discomfort I'm feeling.

What I've observed is that it never actually helps. It just makes my nervous system more frazzled and the thoughts even louder. The escape becomes another trap.

You don't need to be addicted to your phone for this to affect you. Here are some signs your brain might be overstimulated:

- You feel uncomfortable in silence or boredom.
- You reach for your phone without thinking.
- You constantly switch between apps or tabs.
- You scroll late at night even when you're tired.
- You feel "fried" or foggy by midafternoon.

When our nervous system never gets a break, it stays in low-grade fight-or-flight mode. That makes it much harder to feel grounded, calm, or connected to our tools.

Creating Digital Boundaries

This isn't about becoming a minimalist monk who throws their phone in the ocean. It's about designing your digital world to support your recovery instead of sabotaging it.

Here are a few practices that can help:

- Use app timers or screen-time limits.
- Delete apps that cause you to spiral or compare.
- Unfollow accounts on social media platforms that are feeding OCD compulsions.
- Charge your phone outside your bedroom.
- Do a morning routine before looking at your phone.
- Take twenty-four-hour social media breaks regularly.

Even a small reduction in digital noise can make a *huge* difference in your mental clarity.

Key Takeaway

We don't have to quit the internet, but we do have to protect our brain. If your world is constantly loud, OCD will be too. Less noise equals more clarity. That's how we give our tools the space to work.

34

SUPPORT SYSTEM

*OCD recovery is personal, but it
doesn't have to be lonely.*

OCD can feel incredibly isolating.

OCD convinces us that our thoughts are shameful. That we're the only ones dealing with this. That no one could possibly understand. When we believe that, we start to withdraw, and we suffer in silence. This is what happened to me.

I still vividly remember the day I found out a colleague at work had OCD. I was shocked that someone else out there was dealing with what I thought made me uniquely broken. Yet the truth is that there are millions of us around the world walking this same path. We don't have to do this alone.

In fact, having the right support system can be one of the most important factors in long-term recovery.

What a Support System Is Not

Let's start by clearing up a common misconception: A support system is *not* someone who reassures you every time you feel anxious. It's not someone who helps you complete compulsions. It's not someone who tries to logic your OCD away.

In fact, if your support person becomes a source of constant reassurance, they may unintentionally be keeping you stuck in the cycle.

What a Support System Is

A healthy support system does the following:

- Validates our experience without feeding our compulsions
- Encourages us to use our tools, even when it's hard
- Gives us space to feel discomfort without rushing in to fix it
- Celebrates our progress and reminds us of how far we've come
- Knows how OCD works and doesn't take our fears at face value

Your support system could be a therapist, coach, friend, partner, parent, or group of people. What matters is that they help us stay grounded in the truth that we're not broken, and we're not alone.

Finding Your People

If you don't feel like you have a strong support system right now, that's okay. It's never too late to build one.

Here are a few places to start:

- Therapists and coaches who specialize in OCD

- Support groups—online or in person
- Friends or family members who are open to learning and supporting without enabling

You deserve people in your corner who lift you up—and who remind you that your thoughts don't define you.

Key Takeaway

OCD thrives in isolation. Recovery thrives in connection. Find your people and let them walk beside you. Not because you can't do it alone—but because you don't *have to.*

35

SACRED PACE

Recovery isn't a race. It's a rhythm.

We live in a culture that glorifies speed, hustle, and achievement. For many of us with OCD, that pressure to keep moving becomes its own compulsion. We're constantly trying to outpace our thoughts, fill our schedules, and distract ourselves from the discomfort.

But healing doesn't happen at breakneck speed.

It happens at a rhythm of life that feels manageable. That's what I call *sacred pace*—a lifestyle rhythm that is sustainable, grounding, and aligned with long-term recovery.

What Sacred Pace Looks Like

- You're not rushing from one thing to the next.
- You build space into your day to be with your brain without distracting yourself.

- You listen to your nervous system and slow down when needed.
- You prioritize quality over quantity.
- You treat recovery like a relationship, not a sprint.

Sacred pace means honoring your energy, your boundaries, and your recovery needs, even when the world around you tells you to speed up.

What It's Not

- It's not laziness.
- It's not avoidance.
- It's not about doing less because you can't handle life.

Sacred pace is about choosing to live *intentionally*. It's about recovering in a way that lasts.

OCD will often tell us that we can't stop. That if we slow down, we'll fall apart. That we need to do more to stay in control.

What I've learned is that more isn't always better.

Sometimes slowing down is the most courageous thing we can do.

Key Takeaway

Healing doesn't come from rushing. It comes from rhythm.

Create a pace you can sustain that supports your long-term recovery.

Call to Action

Find Your Sacred Pace

Take a moment to reflect on one area of your life that feels rushed, overloaded, or out of balance. What's one small change you could make this week to slow down and create a more sacred, sustainable pace for your long-term recovery? Bonus points if it's in alignment with your values.

36

NUTRITION AND OCD

FUEL FOR RECOVERY

Why Nutrition Matters

You've probably heard that "food is fuel," but when you're dealing with OCD, food is more than just fuel. It's one of the tools that can help stabilize our mood, manage anxiety, and support our brain and body through recovery.

Our brains are constantly working—processing thoughts, regulating emotions, and keeping us alert for threats (real or imagined). Without proper nutrition, the brain gets depleted faster. Low blood sugar, big sugar crashes, or skipping meals can leave us feeling "hangry," foggy, and more vulnerable to intrusive thoughts.

I learned this the hard way. During some of my worst OCD spikes, I was skipping meals, relying on coffee, and eating whatever was fastest—not what was best for my recovery. When I finally started paying attention to how I was fueling my body, I noticed my baseline anxiety started to drop. I wasn't "cured," but the floor wasn't falling out from under me every afternoon.

What to Eat for a Calmer Brain

You don't need a perfect diet (in fact, chasing perfection is an OCD trap). What matters most is eating in a way that supports your energy, focus, and overall well-being.

Focus on these elements:

- **Protein with every meal:** Have eggs, chicken, fish, tofu, legumes, or nuts/seeds. Protein helps keep blood sugar stable and supports neurotransmitter production.
- **Healthy fats:** Incorporate avocado, olive oil, nuts, seeds, or fatty fish. These support brain health and reduce inflammation.
- **Plenty of fiber:** Get your veggies, fruits, beans, and whole grains—fiber supports gut health, which is closely connected to mood and anxiety.
- **Regular meals/snacks:** Don't go more than four to five hours without eating. This helps keep blood sugar—and mood—more stable.

What to Minimize

- **Refined sugars and processed foods:** They can spike blood sugar, then crash it, leading to irritability and more anxiety.
- **Skipping meals or extreme diets:** These can backfire, leaving you depleted and more prone to intrusive thoughts.
- **Too much caffeine or energy drinks:** These can spike anxiety, especially on an empty stomach.

As an example, I remember one morning eating pancakes drenched in maple syrup. Within thirty minutes, my heart was pounding, and I felt lightheaded. At first, I couldn't figure out why I was suddenly anxious. Then I realized what I'd eaten: sugar.

That moment was just one of hundreds that taught me how my blood sugar affects my mood. I've since modified my diet to stay more balanced throughout the day, and it's made a huge difference in my energy and mental clarity. It's not that I won't ever eat pancakes with syrup again, but I'll be more mindful about how much and understand the trade-offs.

Perfectionism and Nutrition

OCD loves to turn healthy habits into rigid rules. If you find yourself obsessing over "eating clean," panicking about food labels, or feeling guilt for eating something "off-plan," take a step back. Nutrition is about nourishment, not punishment. It's okay if you don't eat perfectly and occasionally indulge in foods that bring you joy but aren't necessarily healthy.

Real Life: How I Eat Now

These days, I keep things simple:

- I aim for protein with every meal.
- I eat regular snacks—especially before big work days or stressful events.
- I batch-cook a few meals on Sundays to make healthy choices easier during the week.
- I don't panic if I have pizza, ice cream, or a donut. That's life, not failure.

Quick, Recovery-Friendly Snack Ideas

- Greek yogurt with berries and nuts
- Whole-grain toast with almond butter and banana
- Chicken or chickpea salad wrap

- Hummus and veggie sticks
- Hard-boiled eggs and fruit
- Protein smoothie with greens, seeds, and frozen berries

The Gut-Brain Connection

What we eat doesn't just feed our body; it feeds our mind.

Probiotics (like those found in yogurt, kefir, and fermented foods) and prebiotics (fiber-rich veggies) can support a healthy gut, which in turn supports mood and anxiety regulation.

If you want to supplement, talk to your doctor or nutritionist first—especially if you have allergies or sensitivities or if you're taking medication.

Key Takeaway

You don't have to be perfect.

Small, consistent changes in how we fuel our body can have a big impact on how we feel, think, and recover. Treat nutrition as one more tool in your recovery toolbox. Something you get to use, not something you have to obsess over.

Call to Action

Make a Small Change

Take a minute to reflect: What's one simple nutrition change you can try this week to support your recovery? Write it down and give yourself credit for showing up.

37

YOUR LIFESTYLE BLUEPRINT

*We can't control our thoughts,
but we can design our lives.*

By now, you've learned that OCD recovery isn't just about what happens in our mind. It's about the way we live.

Recovery doesn't happen by accident; it happens by design.

This chapter is here to help you zoom out and look at the big picture—to take everything we've discussed in this section and begin crafting your own lifestyle blueprint for long-term healing.

The Core Pillars

Here are the foundational areas we've explored:

- **Sleep:** Prioritize seven to nine hours and use nighttime routines, supplements, and a consistent wind-down time.

- **Exercise:** Move your body regularly to balance your nervous system, not punish it.
- **Meditation:** Build the muscle to observe your thoughts, not react to them.
- **Nutrition:** Fuel your brain with steady energy throughout the day.
- **Supplements:** Use targeted support to reduce baseline anxiety (if helpful and approved by your provider).
- **Substances:** Mindfully manage alcohol, caffeine, cannabis, and nicotine.
- **Digital hygiene:** Reduce overstimulation and give your brain space to breathe.
- **Nature:** Reconnect with the outdoors to ground your body and mind.
- **Support system:** Surround yourself with people who understand OCD and support your growth.
- **Sacred pace:** Create a rhythm of life that sustains you rather than depletes you.

Build Your Blueprint

Here's a simple exercise to pull it all together:

1. Rate yourself 1 to 5 in each category above (1 = needs serious attention, 5 = solid and supportive).
2. Pick one area you want to focus on first.
3. Create a micro-goal for that area (e.g., "Walk for ten minutes after lunch three times a week" or "Charge my phone outside the bedroom three nights a week").
4. Track your progress for thirty days.
5. Reassess, tweak, and build momentum.

The goal isn't perfection but consistency. And your lifestyle blueprint doesn't have to look like anyone else's. It just has to support the recovery you want.

Key Takeaway

Recovery happens in layers, and our lifestyle is the foundation. If our lifestyle is chaotic, our mind will be chaotic and OCD symptoms will intensify.

We don't need a perfect lifestyle, but we need a supportive one. While we can't control our thoughts, we *can* design our life around our healing.

Take the Next Step with OCD Space

OCD Space is a digital recovery platform where you can work with Oscar, our clinically trained AI OCD coach, 24/7. Oscar will help guide you through OCD recovery so you can keep making progress anytime, anywhere.

Join OCDspace.com and start working with Oscar today

PART 7

STAYING FREE

38

WHAT RECOVERY REALLY LOOKS LIKE

*Healing doesn't mean never struggling
again. It means knowing what to
do when you do.*

If you've made it this far, I hope you've started to realize something: Recovery isn't about getting rid of all your intrusive thoughts. It's not about eliminating anxiety forever. It's not about perfection.

Recovery is about freedom.

Freedom to live your life without compulsions running the show. Freedom to feel anxious without needing to fix it. Freedom to think random thoughts and keep going. Most importantly, freedom to respond to OCD on *your* terms.

Recovery Isn't Linear

One of the biggest traps we OCDers fall into is expecting recovery to be a straight line. We'll be doing great, then *bam*—a new trigger, a tough week, a dip in energy, and suddenly OCD is loud again.

This doesn't mean we've failed or reverted to square one. It means we're human.

OCD recovery happens in layers, like peeling an onion. We make progress, we hit a new layer, we apply our tools, and we grow again. Each round teaches us more and deepens our trust in ourselves.

Here's what lasting recovery includes:

- Intrusive thoughts still showing up from time to time
- Discomfort still rising when you're triggered
- OCD trying to change themes or sneak in sideways
- Days when your tools feel harder to use
- Moments when you think, "Am I back at square one?"

Here's the difference: Now, you know what's happening, and you have the tools. You don't spiral for weeks anymore; you bounce back faster.

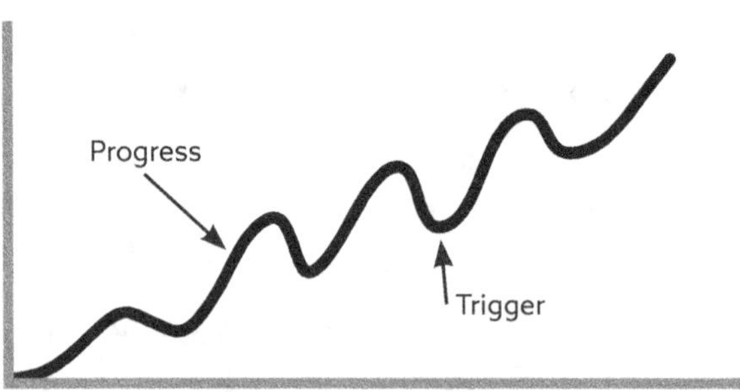

Mindset Reminder

A Flare-Up Isn't Failure

Recovery isn't linear. A hard day (or week or month) doesn't mean you're back at square one. Trust the process. Come back to the basics. And most importantly—just do today.

Key Takeaway

Freedom doesn't come from eliminating OCD. It comes from changing your relationship with it. The thoughts may still come, but now you know how to meet them and stay free.

39

YOUR RECOVERY PLAN

You don't need motivation.
You need a system.

The hardest part of recovery isn't knowing what to do—it's consistently doing it.

You've come a long way in this book. You've learned how OCD works, how to stop feeding the cycle, how to apply the four core responses, how to do ERP, how to utilize letting go, and how to optimize your brain and body.

Now it's time to build a plan that brings it all together. Because when the intrusive thoughts hit, and they will, it's not about motivation. It's about having a system you can fall back on.

Step 1: Know Your Pattern

Take some time to write this out:

- What are your most common intrusive thoughts or themes?

- What compulsions do you typically do (mental or physical)?
- What does a typical OCD spiral look like for you?

Awareness is power. When you know your patterns, you can interrupt them sooner with the tools you've learned throughout this book.

Step 2: Lock In Your Tools

Pick the tools that resonate most:

- The four core responses (acceptance, uncertainty, indifference, agreement)
- The letting go technique
- ERP (in vivo, scripting)
- Sacred pace
- Meditation
- Your support system

You don't need to use everything every day, but you do need to know what works for you.

Step 3: Build Your Routine

Recovery isn't something you remember to do. It's something you *build into your life.*

Ask yourself these questions:

- What's my morning routine?
- When do I meditate or move my body?
- When do I plan exposure work?
- How do I wind down?

Even just ten to twenty minutes a day of intentional practice can change your life. The goal isn't to do more; it's to do what matters *consistently*.

Key Takeaway

Recovery isn't about doing everything perfectly. It's about doing the helpful things regularly.

You have what you need. You've built awareness. You've practiced the tools. Now it's time to commit to a plan that helps you stay free. Let this be the start of your next chapter.

FINAL WORDS

This isn't the end. It's your beginning.

When I was diagnosed with OCD in 2016, I truly thought my life was over.

I believed I was doomed to suffer forever, that I'd never feel peace. I thought I'd never be myself again. The thoughts felt too loud and too dark. I didn't know what was happening, and I had no idea there were tools that could help.

But I kept going.

I found the right support. I learned the tools. I practiced them day after day—often when it felt pointless, uncomfortable, and like I was getting nowhere.

Then something amazing happened: My life got better. Not perfect or thought-free, but better than I thought was possible.

Since then, I've written books. Founded companies. Climbed Mount Kilimanjaro with my dad. I married the woman of my dreams. I live a life I used to think was impossible.

This is not because OCD disappeared; it's because I stopped letting it be in charge.

If I can do it, so can you.

If you've made it to the end of this book, that tells me something important: You're willing, and you're ready.

My advice? Block out the next ninety days and make recovery your top priority.

Use this book as your guide. Pair it with therapy or coaching. Show up daily with compassion and courage.

Go all-in because the future version of you will be so glad you did.

I'm wishing you all the strength and self-compassion in the world as you continue your journey.

Take the Next Step with OCD Space

You don't need to have this all figured out right now.

Recovery doesn't come from understanding everything perfectly—it comes from practicing, again and again, how you respond when OCD shows up.

If you want support applying what you've learned here in real life, Oscar, our clinically trained AI OCD coach, is there to help you slow things down, see the cycle more clearly, and choose a recovery-aligned response in the moments that matter most.

You can start your free trial anytime at OCDspace.com

RESOURCES AND WAYS TO GET INVOLVED

You're not alone, and you don't have to do this alone.

Whether you're looking for deeper support, community, or educational tools, here are several powerful resources to support your journey.

OCDspace.com—Your 24/7 Digital Recovery Platform

OCD Space is a comprehensive online platform designed to support you at every stage of your recovery. At its core is **Oscar**, our clinically trained AI OCD coach, available 24/7 to guide you through proven strategies like ERP, the letting go technique, and the 4 Core Responses.

Whether you're working through a challenging spike, building your exposure hierarchy, or looking for encouragement in between therapy sessions, OCD Space gives you the tools, structure, and guidance you need—anytime, anywhere.

Think of Oscar as your recovery companion, helping you stay consistent, track your progress, and put the concepts from this book into action in your daily life.

<table><tr><td>

Important

*OCD Space is **not** a replacement for therapy, diagnosis, or treatment by a licensed mental health professional. It's a recovery support tool designed to complement your existing care plan.*

Learn more and get started at OCDspace.com

</td></tr></table>

OCD-Focused Organizations

These organizations are doing powerful work in the OCD industry—whether through research, education, or support:

- **International OCD Foundation (IOCDF):** iocdf.org
- **NOCD:** treatmyocd.com
- **One Mind:** onemind.org
- **Made of Millions:** madeofmillions.com

Recommended Reading

Here are five evidence-based, recovery-forward books we trust:

- *The Mindfulness Workbook for OCD* by Jon Hershfield and Tom Corboy
- *Freedom from Obsessive-Compulsive Disorder* by Jonathan Grayson
- *Brain Lock* by Jeffrey M. Schwartz
- *Everyday Mindfulness for OCD* by Jon Hershfield and Shala Nicely
- *Rewire Your Anxious Brain* by Catherine M. Pittman and Elizabeth M. Karle

Each of these books complements the tools in this one, whether you're just starting or reinforcing your recovery.

Spread the Word

If this book helped you, please leave a five-star rating and review on Amazon. Consider sharing it with someone who might be struggling. You never know who might need the message that recovery is possible.

OTHER TREATMENT CONSIDERATIONS

TMS: A New Frontier in OCD Treatment

While medication has been a standard option for treating OCD for decades, there's another tool that's gaining more traction. It's called *transcranial magnetic stimulation*, or *TMS*. For some of us OCDers, it's been a game changer.

What Is TMS?

TMS is a non-invasive, FDA-approved treatment that uses magnetic pulses to stimulate specific areas of the brain—particularly the ones involved in OCD, anxiety, and mood regulation.

Most often, the treatment targets the anterior cingulate cortex, pre-supplementary motor area (pre-SMA), and dorsomedial prefrontal cortex, which are linked to overactive error detection and obsessive thinking.

Sessions are done in-office, usually five days a week for six to eight weeks. You sit in a chair while a device delivers pulses to your scalp. There's no anesthesia, no downtime, and you're awake the entire session.

What the Research Says

Clinical studies have shown that TMS can reduce the severity of OCD symptoms, especially in OCDers who haven't responded well to medication or therapy alone.

It doesn't "cure" OCD, but it may quiet the noise long enough to help you do the deeper work. Like medication, it's not a replacement for ERP or mindset tools. It's a *supportive tool* that can give you some space to apply what you're learning.

Who TMS Might Be For

TMS is worth exploring if any of the below apply to you:

- You've tried multiple medications and haven't found relief.
- You're dealing with intense OCD symptoms that make ERP feel out of reach.
- You want a nonmedication alternative with clinical support.
- You're looking for options beyond talk therapy or coaching alone.

Talk to your psychiatrist or a local TMS clinic to learn whether you're a good fit. Not everyone qualifies, but if you do, it's worth considering.

What I've Heard from the Community

I've spoken with people in our community who've gone through TMS. Here's what they say:

- "It gave me just enough relief to start doing ERP more consistently."
- "It didn't make the thoughts disappear, but I wasn't as scared of them anymore."

- "TMS helped bring my nervous system down to a level where the mindset tools could finally stick."

Like everything else in this book, this is not a magic fix. It's a promising option, especially if you're feeling stuck and need more support.

Psychedelics and OCD: What We Know So Far

In the last few years, psychedelics like psilocybin and ketamine have reentered the spotlight, not as party drugs but as potential treatments for mental health conditions, including OCD. They're not a replacement for doing the work, but they *might* play a supportive role for some people, in the right context.

Let's unpack what we know so far.

Psilocybin

Psilocybin is the active compound found in certain species of psychedelic mushrooms. Early research shows that when used under controlled, clinical conditions, psilocybin-assisted therapy may help reduce obsessive thinking and increase psychological flexibility.

In these studies, participants often describe gaining a sense of detachment from their thoughts, seeing things with new perspective, or feeling more emotionally open to the thoughts and feelings, which make it easier to engage in ERP and let go of compulsions.

The psilocybin itself did not get rid of thoughts, but it helped the user feel more accepting of the thoughts.

The reality is that psilocybin is still experimental for OCD, however. It's not FDA-approved (yet) and is currently being researched in controlled trials.

This is not something to try on your own or without professional guidance.

Ketamine

Unlike psilocybin, ketamine is already FDA-approved as an anesthetic, and in recent years, it's been repurposed as a rapid-acting treatment for depression, anxiety, and OCD in some clinics.

Ketamine is often administered via infusion, nasal spray (like Spravato), or lozenge. Some people report that it helps create a brief reduction in obsessive thought loops, giving them a window to apply the tools from ERP or therapy more effectively.

Still, like psilocybin, it's not a stand-alone solution. It's not a cure.

Important Notice

I am not a licensed medical professional, and nothing in this section should be considered medical advice.

If you're considering psychedelic-assisted therapy or TMS, talk to a licensed provider—ideally, someone familiar with OCD and trauma-informed practices. Psychedelics can bring up intense emotional experiences and should always be approached with care.

Key Takeaway

None of these options are a replacement for the work and tools discussed throughout this book, but they may serve as support for the work.

If you've been struggling to get traction with traditional treatment, these options could be the extra layer that helps you move forward.

OCD DOESN'T ALWAYS TRAVEL ALONE

You are not broken. You're human.
And you're not alone in this.

It's common to assume OCD is the only thing we're dealing with, until we realize that there's more going on under the surface.

In reality, OCD often shows up with other health conditions. That doesn't mean you're doing something wrong. It means you're human, and you're navigating a complex nervous system that's doing its best to protect you.

Co-Occurring Conditions

Here are some of the conditions that can show up alongside OCD:

- **Generalized anxiety disorder (GAD):** This is ongoing, excessive worry that isn't always tied to a specific obsession.
- **Depression:** This involves feelings of hopelessness, fatigue, low motivation, and emotional numbness.

- **ADHD:** This creates difficulty focusing, impulsivity, or executive functioning challenges that can complicate ERP or mindset work.
- **Body dysmorphic disorder (BDD):** This is a preoccupation with perceived flaws in appearance, often paired with repetitive checking or avoidance behaviors.
- **Eating disorders:** This involves compulsions around food restriction, control, or binge-and-purge cycles, sometimes overlapping with contamination or "just right" OCD.
- **Trichotillomania (hairpulling) and dermatillomania (skin picking):** These body-focused repetitive behaviors bring momentary relief but increase shame or distress.
- **Schizo-OCD:** This involves intrusive thoughts about losing touch with reality, developing schizophrenia, or "going crazy." These fears often feel uniquely terrifying.

"But What If I Develop One of These?"

This is a common theme in OCD: "What if I develop depression?" or "What if I snap and get schizophrenia?" or "What if I already have something worse and don't know it?"

Let's be clear: That's still OCD talking. It's just another attempt to pull you into the OCD cycle. The tools don't change. You meet that fear with the same core responses:

- "Maybe I will, maybe I won't."
- "It is what it is."
- "This thought is allowed to be here."

You don't need a new protocol. You need to keep doing the work you've been doing.

What to Do If You Suspect a Co-Occurring Condition

If you resonate with one of the conditions listed above, consider working with a licensed therapist or psychiatrist who has experience with both OCD and co-occurring disorders. Doing so doesn't mean you're failing. It just means you're getting the full support you deserve. And the good news? The tools in this book still work.

Whether it's ERP, the four core responses, the letting go technique, or lifestyle optimization—these tools can help regulate your system no matter how layered your experience is.

Key Takeaway

OCD doesn't always travel alone. You're not broken, and you're not behind. You're a person navigating real stuff, and you're doing the work.

You've got this.

ACKNOWLEDGMENTS

This book, and the recovery journey it represents, would not exist without the love, support, and guidance of some truly incredible people.

To my wife: You are my rock. Thank you for standing by me, believing in me, and walking every step of this healing journey with me. Your love has grounded me more than words can express.

To my family and close friends: Thank you for your support, encouragement, and unwavering belief in me, even in the moments when I didn't believe in myself.

To 2X: Thank you for helping me step into the next version of myself, not just as a creator and business owner but as a leader and visionary. Your mentorship reshaped what I believed was possible.

To Joseph Moheban: Your guidance, friendship, and support have been pivotal over this decade-long journey. Thank you for always being there when I needed it.

To Lindsey: Your talent as a copy editor, your partnership in launching this project, and your support have been invaluable.

To Greg: Thank you for believing in the mission and for connecting the dots that brought key people together. You helped light the spark that became OCD Space.

To Yash: Your kindness, brilliance, and strategic vision helped bring OCD Space to life. I'm deeply grateful for your hard work, care, and commitment to building something that genuinely helps people.

To Carly Samach: Thank you for your generosity and clinical expertise. Your thoughtful feedback throughout this journey has helped sharpen and elevate this work in ways I deeply appreciate.

To Chris Leins: Thank you for your unwavering focus on OCD Space and on the mission behind it. Your commitment to helping people around the world better understand and recover from OCD has shaped this work in ways that matter. I'm deeply grateful for your focus, integrity, and belief in what we're building.

And finally—to every person who's trusted me with their story, utilized OCD Space, or taken a single brave step toward recovery: This book is for you. You are proof that freedom is possible.

ABOUT ZACH WESTERBECK

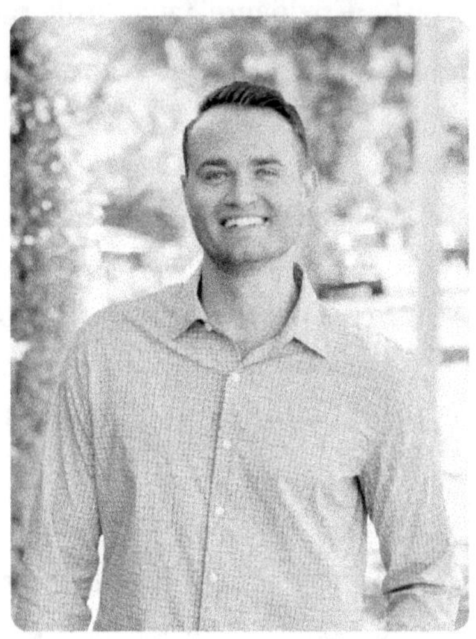

Zach Westerbeck is the founder of **OCD Space**. He's also a husband and father.

Zach is an outspoken advocate for OCD education and recovery. Since being diagnosed with OCD in 2016, he's made it his life's work to make the tools of recovery more accessible, personal, and effective for the millions of people struggling in silence.

He's built a global platform with thousands of followers across Instagram, creating recovery-focused content that reduces stigma, inspires hope, and teaches OCD recovery skills.

Through digital tools, public speaking, and online content, Zach helps people reclaim their lives from OCD using practical strategies rooted in lived experience, neuroscience, exposure therapy, and deep mindset work.

His mission is simple: to bring resources to the more than **350 million people worldwide** living with OCD so they can live freer, more joyful lives.

ENDNOTES

Chapter 4

1   World Health Organization, "Depression and Other Common Mental Disorders: Global Health Estimates," 2017, https://www.who.int/publications/i/item/depression-global-health-estimates.

2   Adam S. Radomsky et al., "Part of a Complete Breakfast: The Presence of Intrusive Thoughts in the Non-Clinical Population," *Journal of Obsessive-Compulsive and Related Disorders* 3, no. 3 (2014) 10.1016/j.jocrd.2013.09.002.

3   Rosemary Banting and Susannah Lloyd, "A Case Study Integrating CBT with Narrative Therapy Externalizing Techniques with a Child with OCD: How to Flush Away the Silly Gremlin," *Journal of Child and Adolescent Psychiatric Nursing* 30, no. 2 (2017): 80–89, https://doi.org/10.1111/jcap.12173. David Epston and Michael White, *Narrative Means to Therapeutic Ends* (W. W. Norton & Company, 1990).

Chapter 5

4   K. Dunlop, B. Woodside, M. Olmsted, P. Colton, P. Giacobbe, and J. Downar, "Reductions in Cortico-Striatal Hyperconnectivity Are Associated with Treatment Response to Dorsomedial Prefrontal Cortex Repetitive Transcranial Magnetic Stimulation in Obsessive-Compulsive Disorder," *Neuropsychopharmacology*, 41(5), 1395–1403. https://doi.org/10.1038/npp.2015.292.

5   Abhishek Purty et al., "Genetics of Obsessive-Compulsive Disorder," *Indian Journal of Psychiatry* 61, suppl. 1 (2019): S37–S42, https://doi.org/10.4103/psychiatry.IndianJPsychiatry_518_18.

Chapter 17

6   J. E. LeDoux, "Emotion Circuits in the Brain," *Annual Review of Neuroscience* 23, no. 1 (2000): 155–84, https://doi.org/10.1146/annurev.neuro.23.1.155. C. S. Carter et al., "Anterior Cingulate Cortex, Error Detection, and the Online Monitoring of Performance," *Science* 280, no. 5364 (1998): 747–49, https://doi.org/10.1126/science.280.5364.747. Jessica Calzà et al., "Altered Cortico-Striatal Functional Connectivity During Resting State in Obsessive-Compulsive Disorder," *Frontiers in Psychiatry* 10 (2019), https://doi.org/10.3389/fpsyt.2019.00319.

7   Ryan J. Jacoby and Jonathan S. Abramowitz, "Inhibitory Learning Approaches to Exposure Therapy: A Critical Review and Translation to Obsessive-Compulsive

Disorder," *Clinical Psychology Review* 49 (2016): 28–40, https://doi.org/10.1016/j.cpr.2016.07.001.

Chapter 19

8   Todd E. Pressman, *Deconstructing Anxiety: The Journey from Fear to Fulfillment* (Rowman & Littlefield, 2019).

Chapter 22

9   David R. Hawkins, *Letting Go: The Pathway of Surrender* (Hay House, 2014).

Chapter 26

10   Nathaniel F. Watson et al., "Recommended Amount of Sleep for a Healthy Adult: A Joint Consensus Statement of the American Academy of Sleep Medicine and Sleep Research Society," *Journal of Clinical Sleep Medicine* 11(6): (2015): 591–92, https://doi.org/10.5664/jcsm.4758.

11   Max Hirshkowitz et al., "National Sleep Foundation's Sleep Time Duration Recommendations: Methodology and Results Summary," *Sleep Health* 1, no. 1 (2015): 40–43, https://doi.org/10.1016/j.sleh.2014.12.010.

12   Irshaad O. Ebrahim et al., "Alcohol and Sleep I: Effects on Normal Sleep," *Alcohol Clinical & Experimental Research* 37, no. 4 (2013): 539–49, https://doi.org/10.1111/acer.12006.

13   Kimberly A. Babson et al., "Cannabis, Cannabinoids, and Sleep: A Review of the Literature," *Current Psychiatry Reports* 19, no. 23 (2017): https://doi.org/10.1007/s11920-017-0775-9.

Chapter 27

14   Harvard Health Publishing, "Exercise Is an All-Natural Treatment to Fight Depression," *Harvard Health*, updated February 2, 2021, https://www.health.harvard.edu/mind-and-mood/exercise-is-an-all-natural-treatment-to-fight-depression.

Chapter 28

15   Harvard Health, "Benefits of Mindfulness," HelpGuide.org, updated January 16, 2025, www.helpguide.org/harvard/benefits-of-mindfulness.htm.

16   "The Science-Backed Benefits of Meditation," Headspace, updated 2020, https://www.headspace.com/science/meditation-research. "Health Benefits of Meditation," Mindworks, accessed 2014, https://mindworks.org/blog/health-benefits-of-meditation/.

Chapter 29

17 Gregory N. Bratman et al, "Nature Experience Reduces Rumination and Subgenual Prefrontal Cortex Activation," *Proceedings of the National Academy of Sciences* 112, no. 28 (2015): 8567–8572, https://doi.org/10.1073/pnas.1510459112.

18 Johann Hari, *Lost Connections: Why You're Depressed and How to Find Hope* (Bloomsbury, 2018).

Chapter 30

19 M. Nematizadeh, H. Ghorbanzadeh, H. S. Moghaddam, M. Shalbafan, M. Boroon, A. A. Keshavarz-Akhlaghi, and S. Akhondzadeh "L-theanine Combination Therapy with Fluvoxamine in Moderate-to-Severe Obsessive-Compulsive Disorder: A Placebo-Controlled, Double-Blind, Randomized Trial," *Psychiatry and Clinical Neurosciences* 77, no. 9:478–85, doi: 10.1111/pcn.13565.

20 Timothy G. Dinan et al., "Psychobiotics: A Novel Class of Psychotropic," *Biological Psychiatry* 74, no. 10 (2013): 720–26, https://doi.org/10.1016/j.biopsych.2013.05.001.

21 B. Dell'Osso et al., "Adjunctive Use of Omega-3 Fatty Acids in Recurrent Depression: A Double-Blind, Placebo-Controlled Study," *Journal of Clinical Psychiatry* 67, no. 5 (2006), 715–22.

22 H. M. Soyak and Ç. Karakükcü, "Investigation of Vitamin D Levels in Obsessive-Compulsive Disorder," *Indian Journal of Psychiatry* 64, no. 4:349–53, doi: 10.4103/indianjpsychiatry.indianjpsychiatry_26_22.

23 Jon E. Grant et al., "N-Acetylcysteine, a Glutamate Modulator, in the Treatment of Trichotillomania: A Double-Blind, Placebo-Controlled Study," *Archives of General Psychiatry* 66, no. 7 (2009): 756–63, https://doi.org/10.1001/archgenpsychiatry.2009.60.

24 M. Fux et al., "Inositol Treatment of Obsessive-Compulsive Disorder," *American Journal of Psychiatry* 153, no. 9, (1996): 1219–21, https://doi.org/10.1176/ajp.153.9.1219.

25 F. A. Zarrouf et al., "Testosterone and Depression: Systematic Review and Meta-Analysis," *Journal of Psychiatric Practice* 15, no. 4 (2009): 289–305, https://doi.org/10.1097/01.pra.0000358315.88931.fc.

26 Kimberly Albert et al., "Estradiol Levels Modulate Brain Activity and Negative Responses to Psychosocial Stress Across the Menstrual Cycle," *Psychoneuroendocrinology* 59 (2015): 14–24, https://doi.org/10.1016/j.psyneuen.2015.04.022.

Chapter 32

27 T. Roehrs and T. Roth, "Sleep, Sleepiness, and Alcohol Use," *Alcohol Research and Health* 25, no. 2 (2001): 101–109, https://pubmed.ncbi.nlm.nih.gov/11584549/.

28 Kimberly A. Babson et al., "Cannabis, Cannabinoids, and Sleep: A Review of the Literature," *Current Psychiatry Reports* 19, no. 23 (2017): https://doi.org/10.1007/s11920-017-0775-9.

29 Astrid Nehlig, "Effects of Coffee/Caffeine on Brain Health and Disease: What Should I Tell My Patients?," *Practical Neurology* 16, no. 2 (2016): 89–95, https://doi.org/10.1136/practneurol-2015-001162.

30 Neal L. Benowitz, "Nicotine Addiction," *New England Journal of Medicine* 362, no. 24 (2010): 2295–2303, https://doi.org/10.1056/NEJMra0809890.